THE *complete*
organic pregnancy

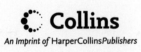

Collins

An Imprint of HarperCollins*Publishers*

THE *complete*
organic pregnancy

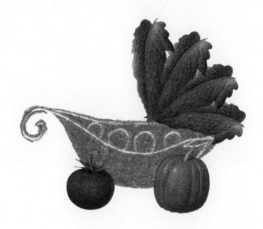

DEIRDRE DOLAN *and* ALEXANDRA ZISSU

Any product mentioned here by name is something we genuinely love and use. We haven't been swayed by freebies, been paid off by CSA farmers, or taken promotional fees from the migratory birds who would prefer you buy shade-grown coffee.

This book is designed to provide information only. It is not intended to be complete or exhaustive, nor is it a substitute for the advice of your physician or other health care professional. You should be under the care of a physician or other health care professional during your entire pregnancy, and should consult that person with respect to all concerns you may have. All efforts have been made to ensure the accuracy of the information contained in this book as of the date published. The author and the publisher expressly disclaim responsibility for any adverse effects arising from the use or application of the information contained herein.

HarperCollins books may be purchased for educational, business, or sales promotional use. For information, please write: Special Markets Department, HarperCollins Publishers, Inc., 10 East 53rd Street, New York, NY 10022.

FIRST EDITION

Designed by Stephanie Huntwork

Library of Congress Cataloging-in-Publication Data has been applied for.

ISBN-10: 0-06-088745-1
ISBN-13: 978-0-06-088745-2

06 07 08 09 10 10 WBC/RRD 10 9 8 7 6 5 4 3 2 1

To Swiss chard

AUTHORS' NOTE

When the time came to get pregnant, one thing was crystal clear for both of us—we wanted our babies to be born as healthy as humanly possible. Because health begins in the womb, we figured our main job was to make sure that ours were pure places to grow. Our first instinct was to eat organic food. It's produced without harmful pesticides or hormones, which would obviously be best for our developing babies. But beyond our diets, we weren't sure what else we could do to make our bodies into the safe havens we wanted them to be.

We're both journalists, so we started doing what we do naturally—asking questions. We cast our nets wide, analyzing the contents of our medicine cabinets, second-guessing everything under our kitchen sinks, even investigating what was in the foam padding of the chairs we were sitting on. We read everything we could (including product labels) and interviewed scientists, chefs, doctors, and farmers. We had always assumed that the people who produce what we eat, use, and wear had our health and safety in mind, and that our government was adequately regulating them. We quickly learned we were wrong to assume anything—particularly when it came to the development of our unborn children. What we discovered was disturbing enough to make us rethink everything from our mattresses to our shower curtains. *The Complete Organic Pregnancy* is the result of that in-depth research.

We've divided the book into the three stages of pregnancy—Part 1: Transitioning, Part 2: Growing, and Part 3: Living. Transitioning is what you want to do before you get pregnant, equal parts purging (good-bye bleach! hello decaf!) and shifting your mind-set. Growing is a nuts-and-bolts guide to the most actively organic pregnancy possible. Living is about the early months with your new baby, and the importance of remaining organic for breastfeeding, health, and the future habits of your family.

An organic pregnancy is about taking environmentalism and personalizing it. It makes sense to think seriously about your baby's first environment—your body. For us, it gives extra meaning to our weekly visit to the farmers' market, our choice to drink out of glass instead of plastic, and the decision to use only nontoxic products to clean. As you'll find, it's an easy lifestyle to embrace. A few basic changes can protect you, your baby, and ultimately the world she'll grow up in. After all, the real heart of our research isn't the big, bad toxins, it's ten delicious fingers and ten equally delectable toes.

Here's to healthy babies.

CONTENTS

PART ONE *transforming*

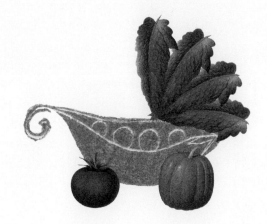

INTRODUCTION

So you're ready to have a baby. If the idea is making you wonder about organic food, and what else you can do to have an organic pregnancy, we're here to tell you what you need to know. We've been there. When we were looking for answers, we couldn't find one definitive resource to rely on. So we decided to create one.

Whether you do 100 percent or any percent of what we suggest here, we believe any organic is better than no organic when it comes to protecting your future baby, yourself, and the environment she will grow up in. Now is the time to purify yourself and your surroundings. There's a lot to consider. The amount of unknown information about the toxins, pesticides, and man-made chemicals that surround us can be overwhelming. We always try to keep in mind, and hope you will, too, that it requires proactivity to steer clear of these dangers. "Everything you avoid is a step in the right direction," says Myra Goodman, founder of Earthbound Farms, the largest grower of organic produce in North America. You're never going to be 100 percent pure or safe. But if you manage just 10 percent, you could avoid the straw that breaks the camel's back. Bodies are meant to deal with a certain amount of toxicity, but we feel like wherever and whenever possible, we'd like to give our babies and ourselves that extra break.

Thinking Beyond Yourself

BY BARBARA KINGSOLVER

I come from a very practical background, a working-class community, where self-indulgence was just not on the ticket, especially for women. In this regard, my upbringing has stayed with me: I'm not the kind of person who could declare that I simply have to have this or that, even when I was pregnant. I recently looked back into my journals to recall my pregnancies, and was surprised to remember that I carried my second child, Lily, through a rigorous book tour during the early months. We hadn't yet announced the pregnancy publicly (and I'm a private person anyway), so I was in no position to ask for special treatment. I just had to be a trooper: eating what I could, when I could, working the long, tough hours, making the next flight on time each day. I remember being very tired and wishing I could go home, mainly so that I could have better control over my food and schedule. But these engagements had been planned for a long time, much longer than I'd been pregnant. So I just did my best.

Obviously, I can relate to every pregnant woman who wishes her life had room in it for a perfect diet, lots of naps, and all kinds of special pampering—but who must live in the real world instead. I always just try to eat the simplest, freshest food I can get, wherever I am, so when I had to grab quick meals on the road, that would have meant a lot of restaurant salad bars, piling on the broccoli for extra calcium. I didn't eat feedlot meat or dairy products that contain antibiotics and hormones, I'm sure. I've been avoiding those things for a long time, pregnant or not.

But I didn't have the option of a perfectly organic life. I kept my nose out for what seemed healthiest in any moment, and cheered myself up by thinking about all the places my baby had secretly sneaked into already. I wrote in my journal, "I'll have to tell this person, once born, that he or she has already shared a stage with Annie Proulx and Jane Smiley, has slipped slender as a knife with me into my black velvet evening gown to entertain the literary lights and dignitaries of Washington, D.C. This clever kid has even been on the *MacNeilLehrer NewsHour,* with no producers the wiser!"

I worked throughout the pregnancy. In the last trimester, I took a long-planned research trip to the Yucatán for a project my husband and I were working on together. I tried to be extra careful about what I ate because we were in some very remote places, often hosted by people who had limited sanitary facilities. I did get sick for a couple of days, but mostly it worked out fine. By then I was quite obviously pregnant, and everyone was sympathetic and helpful. It was a fantastic cultural experience. I was interviewing refugee women living (sometimes quasi-legally) at the edge of a forest preserve, people who had reason to be wary of outsiders, but my great big belly was a wonderful icebreaker. Everybody in Mexico seems to know just what pregnant women need. Lots of fresh eggs and vegetables, lots of weak tea (I was grateful for the boiled water), plenty of advice and congratulations.

Looking back on that trip, I realize that even without my asking for anything special, my pregnancy was an important part of the experience. Working through a pregnancy, living the challenging lives that modern women lead, is not a bad thing. Nor is it a modern thing, of course—women have worked hard through their pregnancies since time began. It's utterly normal, and probably healthier than sitting idle and worrying too much. You just have to bring some extra diligence to the project.

I'll grant that these experiences sound pretty exotic, but basically I had two completely normal pregnancies. These were enjoyable times for me, surprisingly so. I'm kind of obsessive about being productive; what a revelation it was, therefore, to think that even while I slept or sat reading the paper, I was busy manufacturing bones, eyeballs, kidneys! I loved the whole prospect and had a strong sense that things would go well. "I've wanted this baby so much," I wrote in my journal, in the fourth week of my first pregnancy, "I can't possibly see it now as an impostor. I just watch, smiling, as it begins to rearrange the furniture of my body—breasts out here, stomach there, digestion in some forgotten corner. Such a tiny guest, to be so bossy."

I did the things every responsible pregnant woman does: didn't smoke or drink alcohol or go hang-gliding. Attended to my needs for extra protein, calcium, and folic acid. I don't like taking vitamins, so whenever I could cook and control my diet, I got what I needed from whole foods. Lots of dark green, leafy vegetables and so forth. I did not have the option of buying exclusively organic ingredients, though there was a big difference between my pregnancies in this regard. I had Camille, my first, in 1987, and Lily in '96—that was a different decade. Products like hormone-free dairy were available by then, even in ordinary grocery stores. If I could honor only one priority for the pregnant diet, it would be to avoid foods containing antibiotics and growth hormones. A lot of pediatricians agree with me on that one.

Pregnancy is a time of eating mindfully—doing a lot of things mindfully, in fact, with acute awareness of the body's new job as a caretaker. It's pretty easy for any of us casually to ignore our bodies' needs, I suppose, but casually abusing a child is quite another matter. This really hit me during my first pregnancy. In my journal, I see that I made a vow to myself right away to grow up, become a mom now, put away lazy habits like skipping meals (which I often used to do, when I was busy). I found that paying attention to my body and my sen ses usually told me what I needed to know. Eating something immediately whenever I felt hungry, for example, really helped stave off morning sickness.

And my nose! Holy cow, nobody tells you this about pregnancy. All the prenatal folklore says you'll crave weird things at midnight (which I never did), but it never tells you that your gag reflex will take up residence front and center, and that your nose will become the nose of a wild dog, increasing its powers a hundredfold until you can sense people and things—such as beer and cigarettes—that have preceded you through a room by hours or days. This part was not so pleasant, but it seemed profoundly protective. Strong chemicals in paint, in food, in soft drinks, in bank carpets, all became unbearable to my nose. It makes perfect sense. I needed to stay away from toxins, and, boy, I did. I have such sympathy for women who have to spend their pregnancies working in factories or hair salons where chemical smells are ubiquitous. I don't know how they do it—and I know they shouldn't have to.

Pregnancy is a natural time to change your life for the better, and motherhood keeps the changes coming. As I mentioned earlier, I was raised in a culture that didn't encourage women to demand much for themselves. But I found I could ask for the moon, when it came to my kids—from myself, my grocer, and my legislators. I don't mean asking for material things, but demanding a safer, kinder place for us all. Raising kids has made me aware of what a wretchedly extravagant, indulgent society I live in—the big cars, the unnecessary appliances, so much waste. We're consuming so much more than our share of the world's petroleum, even changing the climate, with devastating effects. When you're thinking carefully about teaching your kids right from wrong, stuff like this kind of leers at you.

A healthy diet has come along with many other changes in my life through a steady process of politicization, always connected with my vision of the world I want my kids to be able to grow up into. In our family, our ideas about food are completely integrated with our politics and our spirituality. My dietary choices are not just concerned with the health of my kids, but also the health of kids on the other side of the globe. Using a lot of fossil fuels, supporting the agrochemical monopolies and industrial agriculture—these things poison the air, water, and soil, and steal from a lot of poor people their own capacity to feed themselves. Those bananas in the grocery traveled a long way in a refrigerated hold, guzzling gas the whole way, and the site of their creation somewhere in the tropics displaced subsistence farms for local people. Dousing those folks with plenty of pesticides was also part of the bargain. I can't look at a banana without seeing all these secret, ugly costs to some vulnerable (maybe pregnant) mother in Honduras or Mexico. Though bananas are famously rich in potassium, there are much kinder ways for me to get it. Potatoes, for example, have twice as much.

The way we eat in our family is the way we live in general: we try to avoid excessive consumption. As much as possible, we eat foods that are grown locally, either in our own garden or by farmers we know. We try to make choices that are least extravagant in terms of using up the world's resources. So if the organic apples in the grocery are from New Zealand, I don't buy them. We've found so many great alternatives. Apples are a good example. In the fall we go to an orchard just down the road, buy several bushels at a time, and have an apple holiday. We bought a steam juicer, so we can put up quarts and quarts of juice to drink all winter. We freeze some for pies, store plenty in the root cellar, and make every apple thing we can think of. When cherries on our local trees come ripe next June, we'll do the same.

The apples at our neighborhood orchard, by the way, are not organic. But because I know the farmer, I can ask him questions. He uses dormant oils, not the really toxic stuff that gets under the skin of the fruit. So at home I fill up the kitchen sink with soapy water and give the apples a bath. I feel better about this than participating in the weird, self-indulgent economy of flying "environmentally friendly" apples halfway around the planet in a cloud of jet fumes. I also believe that if we all supported our local farmers, at least a little, this weird economy would change for the better. More organic and local options would become available.

I don't have any hard-and-fast rules. Organic may not always be the best choice, especially what I call "boutique organic"—meaning long-distance imports or the fancy, highly processed (and very expensive) health foods that come as packaged meals and snacks. Convenience food is okay in a pinch, but not as a lifestyle. For me, simplicity is usually the best choice: in food, as in child rearing on the whole. We always tended to skip the complicated toys in favor of books, walks in the woods, pots and pans to bang on. Now that my kids are older, they're very good at entertaining themselves. And they know how to cook, too. Cooking your own food at home is economical, healthy, and the only way to know for sure what's going into your mouth. If you're ever going to give up the corn syrup, trans fats, and other awful junk that's in processed foods, pregnancy is a fine time to start.

When someone has taken up residence in your belly, you're forced to slow down and think beyond yourself. First, of your own baby. Then someone else's. The motherhood chemicals start to swim around in your brain, and the next thing you know, you've realized something huge about all those kids in Sri Lanka, in Ethiopia, the casualties of war and global warming and our country's endless greediness for resources: every one of those hungry, left-out people is somebody's baby. Every bite you take is part of a larger equation, involving the magical sum called "enough to go around."

BARBARA KINGSOLVER's eleven books include essay collections, short stories, poetry, an oral history, and many well-known novels, including The Bean Trees *and* The Poisonwood Bible. *She and her husband, Steven Hopp, and their two daughters grow most of their own food on a farm in southern Appalachia.*

food

why organic matters

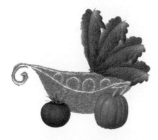

Definitions of the word organic can be technical (see box on next page), but it basically means that crops aren't chemically fertilized or treated with chemical pesticides, and that animals are fed grains produced from pesticide-free crops. Since organic food has grown in popularity, a number of studies have supported its health benefits. To name a few: The 2005 Centers for Disease Control and Prevention's *National Report on Human Exposure to Environmental Chemicals* cites a study that found that preschool-aged children eating organic fruits and vegetables had concentrations of pesticides in their urine six times lower than children eating conventional produce. A 2002 study by the Consumers Union (the publisher of *Consumer Reports*) and Organic Materials Research Institute published in the journal *Food Additives and Contaminants* found that "Organic foods had consistently minimal or nonexistent pesticide residue." Finally, a 1999 study sponsored by the Department of Agriculture found that pastured animals (meaning they can walk around) provide less saturated fat and more nutrients than their factory-raised counterparts.

For a mother-to-be, this knowledge can turn grocery shopping into an empowering experience. Choose organic, and you've already done something good for your baby. Pre-pregnancy is the perfect time to shift your diet and clear your system of toxic food. We'll focus more on which pesticides to avoid and how in Part 2. But before we do we want to suggest that there is more to eating organically than the fact that it's good for you. Ask organophiles why they eat this way, and their answers are often philosophical: They believe that the way they're eating helps not only them, but the farmers who grow their food, and the earth in general. "Organics is about living without harming yourself and your environment," says cookbook author Deborah Madison, founding chef of Greens Restaurant in San Francisco.

On a practical level, choosing organic food over conventional involves some extra effort when shopping, more time in the kitchen (it's harder to eat organically when dining out or ordering in), and sometimes a little more cash. But the best part is, without a middleman, food tastes a whole lot better.

whole foods diet

For us, organic eating doesn't really involve much besides fresh fruits, vegetables, grains, dairy, meat, and sometimes fish. Though you can now buy everything from certified organic frozen burritos to certified organic gummy bears, packaged foods don't provide the same nutritional value as whole foods. This isn't to say those gummy bears (made with organic cane sugar, plus beet and carrot juice to dye them various colors) aren't tasty. But they don't do anything for you. And you want your body in tip-top shape as you try to get pregnant.

We're not going to spell out a strict diet for you to follow. Every person varies in what he or she wants and needs to eat. We've never liked the specific do-and-don't diets in traditional pregnancy books. We'll always insist a whole foods diet is the best way to go, which simply means eating food as close to the form that it came out of the earth as possible. "I don't believe in artificial things, even if they call them organic," says Joan Dye Gussow, former head of the nutrition department at Columbia University and author of *This Organic Life: Confessions of a Suburban Homesteader.* "How can you have a natural margarine? I have always eaten butter." Gussow strongly believes you should eat food that travels the shortest distance from the farmer to you so that you know how your food is being grown.

The word "whole" should be taken literally, too. When possible, we try to think of our chickens as complete birds instead of parts, all of which can be put to some use. Try to take the same approach with carrot tops and celery fronds—if you have time, they make great vegetable stock.

eating organic while trying to conceive

We all have toxins in our bodies. Our theory is this: get out as many as you can now in preparation for your new tenant. Stocking up on as much iron and calcium and folic acid and other good-for-baby food could help during your first trimester, when many women have a hard time stomaching vegetables (or anything for that matter). Cleaning up your act now will also help set up a good, healthy base, as it

THE IMPORTANCE OF FOLIC ACID

Folic acid is a B vitamin used in our bodies to make new cells. Having enough folic acid in your body before you're pregnant helps prevent major birth defects of the brain and spine (known as neural tube defects), which can happen in the first few weeks of pregnancy—often before a woman realizes she is pregnant. It's recommended that all women of childbearing age take a multivitamin containing 400 mg of folic acid daily, in addition to eating a healthy, balanced diet. The CDC suggests eating folic-acid-fortified cereal. Though we take prenatal vitamins (which contain 1,000 mg of folate), we prefer to supplement our folic with sources earthier than fortified packaged products. Try some of these:

Whole wheat (breads, cereals, etc.)
Eggs
Beans (lentils, chickpeas, black, and lima)
Sunflower seeds
Asparagus
Leafy green vegetables
Oranges or orange juice
Strawberries
Cantaloupe and other melons

is harder to change your diet once you start feeling bad. "This is something you have to do for life, for your child, and for forever," says chef Alice Waters, a pioneer of the organic movement. "It's a way of looking at the world and understanding the relationship of food, of health, well-being, culture, and environment."

When shifting your diet to a more organic, whole foods approach, one of the first things to do is to look at the amount of sugar you consume and cut back. These are empty calories, devoid of nutrients. When you're pregnant, you'll want to make sure pretty much everything you consume contains essential nutrients. Sweetened beverages—including fruit juice—are a big source of sugar. So are packaged foods. Get in the habit of reading labels at the supermarket if you don't already. The shorter the ingredient list, the better. If you don't recognize an ingredient, you can look it up, but it's probably not good for you.

Though the sweetener you add to things like tea is negligible compared with what pops up in packaged foods and corn-syrup-filled sodas, choose it wisely. We always thought brown sugar was more nutritious than white. But it turns out that in this country, due to government regulations similar to those for raw milk

- Milk and dairy—Choose organic and items without hormones and antibiotics.
- Meat—Eat lean; bio-accumulating chemicals, pesticides, and toxins get stored in animal fat. Buy organic or at least pastured (see pages 89–93).
- Fruits and veggies—Choose organic when possible. For a list of best and worst conventional fruits and vegetables, see pages 94–96.
- Eat locally and seasonally whenever possible. Peaches don't grow in the fall. Apples do.

cheese, all sugar is first processed to white to clean it, which removes any valuable nutrients. Brown sugar is just white sugar with molasses added back in. Maple syrup isn't much better; it's filtered. Opt for honey when possible (although it should never be given to an infant under one year old). Another reason to avoid high fructose corn syrup is that you never know what pesticides and herbicides the corn was sprayed with, or if the corn was genetically modified.

Toxic Shock

BY LEXY ZISSU

The first time my boyfriend, Olli, and I had deliberate let's-make-a-baby sex was just plain weird. We were still in the talking-about-it phase when it just sort of happened. I lay in bed afterward, freaking out. To my surprise, my panic had very little to do with the idea of a child.

My anxiety was about my physical world, suddenly looming over me. I tried to concentrate on that what-if-we-just-made-something feeling, but the crack in the ceiling above my head distracted me. It was suggesting a different sort of what-if. As in, what if that's lead paint? What if that stain where the window meets the wall is actually toxic mold?

What if the zit cream I smeared on my face before climbing into bed can lead to birth defects? And the wine I drank hours earlier? The fumes wafting through the vents from my building's boiler?

Olli wandered into the bedroom, unfazed, with a glass of water. I sipped. He turned out the lights. I couldn't sleep. Why had I taken a sip? We use a Brita filter. But what if even Brita isn't safe? What's in that filter anyway? The water sits in a plastic pitcher in our fridge. Isn't plastic toxic? And plastic is everywhere—my computer, all of my food storage containers, the television, the printer, the remote control, the Cuisinart, the garbage pail, the hangers, all of the plastic bags, my phone. What about cell phones? Eventually I drifted off.

The next morning I made coffee on autopilot, momentarily forgetting what had happened. I was putting brown sugar into our cups, when I dropped the spoon. The sugar could be deadly! (Not to mention that I shouldn't have been caffeinating.) It was a gift from a close friend in Jamaica, thoughtfully smuggled on a flight to New York. American brown sugar is refined to white with "cleaned" molasses added back in. Jamaican sugar is like French cheese—unprocessed. And now that I was possibly pregnant, the microbe-unfriendly USDA didn't seem so wacky anymore. Maybe those beautiful wet granules contained germs that would harm my unborn kid. I poured my coffee into the sink.

I headed to the shower to calm my nerves. Fat chance. The bathroom was like a House of Horrors. Can Soft Scrub residue get in your system via your feet? What about the black mold dancing across our (plastic!) shower curtain? And the roach bait behind the toilet? The cat litter winked at me; I recoiled. I brushed my teeth and almost cracked—was fluoride bad? And what about my deodorant (aluminum), hydrocortisone cream (steroids), and just about every shampoo, lotion, and perfume on my shelf (all made with chemicals that have the potential to harm growing babies)? Even my pedicure made me nervous, but I didn't dare risk acetone fumes to remove the poisonous polish.

The phone rang—my friend Deirdre. She had been trying for a few months. I broke down: "I've lost my mind. Do you think subway fumes can pickle a kid? I have to quit my job; my chair has stuffing poking out of it. I bet it's toxic. Everyone there has the same cold all the time."

"Okay, Lexy," she said, humoring me. "What are you talking about?"

"We tried last night. The people downstairs smoke cigarettes and pot constantly. It floats up around the heat riser by my pillow. That can't be good."

"My neighbor smokes, too. You can't think like that. If there's something you can do, do it, but you have to live in the world. Can you shut the heat vent? Just write down everything you're freaking out about and we'll start Googling." D's good like that. Trying to get pregnant has made her hyperaware, but she's also a realist.

I started to make breakfast. Scrambled organic eggs with organic scallions (well done, just in case, and not in a nonstick pan, for good measure). I sliced up an organic wheat baguette from my favorite local place. The bread—and Deirdre—soothed me. I used to be this neurotic about everything I ate. Simple newspaper articles would lead me to think lettuce was deadly. As a defense, I researched everything that concerned me and decided eating organic would save my health—and my sanity. I promised Deirdre I'd take the same approach with my cracked ceiling.

Olli climbed out of bed and retrieved the remaining cup of coffee. He smiled. As I sectioned my grapefruit, I didn't feel pregnant. But I knew that by the time I was, I would have figured out if my aluminum grapefruit spoons were out to hurt our offspring. If they were, I've always preferred silver anyway.

the competing wisdom of local versus organic

One thought on a growing and complex debate: long-time supporters of organic food have recently shifted to championing local over organic. This has a lot to do with the desire to eat food that doesn't have to travel thousands of miles on a fuel-filled jet to get to your plate. Joan Dye Gussow, who sat on the National Organic Standards Board for five years, is more committed to local food than she is to organic. "I personally feel that eating organic food from California or Venezuela if you live in New York is not the way to go," says Gussow, who grows most of her own food in her backyard in upstate New York. Not everyone has the opportunity or the time to go quite this far, but she's concerned that if everyone eats food that has to be flown or trucked to them, there will be no local farms left to feed people when fuel prices make long-haul transportation of food prohibitively expensive. The growing number of farmers' markets across the country have made eating local a lot easier to do, especially in growing season. Some small farmers can't afford to get certified as organic, but if you talk to them while perusing their eggplants and tomatoes and ask them how they deal with pest management and what they spray, you'll find many come close to meeting organic standards. The issue isn't black and white. *Vegetarian Cooking for Everyone* author Deborah Madison, for example, would support a small farmer using some spray over having him or her lose an entire orchard to blight, even though this would go against organic standards. Madison lives outside Santa Fe, New Mexico, and also prefers not to buy organic from distant places. She knows most of the farmers at her farmers' market and has personally visited many of their farms. "I think being organic means being an involved person," she says. "You have to ask questions." Alice Waters agrees that it's crucial to support the people who are taking care of the land: "Sustainable farmers want our children to be enriched by a culture that is diverse, and if we don't take care, we're not going to have that." For people interested in local in most parts of the country, winter can present a challenge. One way to deal with this is to buy from farmers who set aside things for the winter, to eat dried foods like beans, and to freeze sauces and fruit during the growing season.

Not all organic enthusiasts are comfortable with going local if it means giving up organic. It's helpful to bear in mind that California-based Earthbound Farms was responsible for keeping over 8 million pounds of agricultural chemicals out of the earth in 2004. The fact is, you vote with your dollars when you choose to buy either local or organic.

cost

Time to tackle the myth that organic food is only for the rich. Yes, it does appear to cost more when you're in the store and see a sign that says NECTARINES: 99¢ A POUND, next to one that says ORGANIC NECTARINES: $2.49 A POUND. But when you start eating a whole foods diet, you cut back drastically on packaged foods. Look at your grocery bill if you don't believe us, but cookies, chips, and frozen meals add up. Many stores that stock organic food also have bulk grain and cereal sections, which can keep prices down. The best way we have found to reduce the cost of organic produce is to join a CSA (Community Supported Agriculture) farm. Some CSAs have meat and fruit; most just have vegetables.

A Year in the Life of Lexy's
Organic Farmer

BY LEXY ZISSU

Faced with two beets—one organic, one conventional—in the aisle of whatever supermarket you frequent, it's not only hard to put the more expensive one in your basket, it's counterintuitive. Why would anyone willingly spend extra? I've trained myself to cough up the cash because I truly know what I'm paying for. But not everyone knows.

The best way I can think to explain why it's worth spending more on organic produce is to introduce my CSA farmer. Which is funny because I spend a lot less on my CSA than I do buying organic produce during the winter. But I want to give you a sense of what it takes to be an organic farmer.

CSA stands for Community Supported Agriculture, which started thirty years ago in Japan and was introduced to the United States in 1985. Members support a farm by purchasing "shares" of the harvest, and pay the farmers before the growing season begins so that they have money to farm the land. I pay a little more than $400 a year for my share in Stoneledge Farm in South Cairo, New York, which is run by Deb and Pete Kavakos. Members receive whatever Deb and Pete harvest weekly, and also share the risk of things like bad weather and crop damage. We get a wide variety of gorgeous, bountiful vegetables that thrive in different conditions delivered to a pickup site in New York City every Tuesday from mid-June to just before Thanksgiving. If money is tight, CSA is the most inexpensive (and wonderful) way of getting organic, local produce. And it's the organic dream—how many people do you know who can say they know the faces behind their lettuce? Once a year Deb and Pete host farm visits. Members head upstate in droves to wander through the fields, pick things, and ask as many questions as they want.

Deb and Pete first got into farming with a home garden years ago when she was pregnant. It progressed from there. When they decided to farm full-time, there was never a question of farming conventionally. Deb describes it as a natural instinct: "I never wanted to have to make excuses for what I do." They also didn't want pesticides and herbicides around their young children. "A farm encompasses your whole life; you're always together; you're always in the soil. It was very important to keep as organic as possible." For a while they had sheep. These days they grow only vegetables. Though they always followed organic standards, they weren't officially certified until 2002. They have been doing CSA almost exclusively in New York for over ten years (though they do sell at two small farmers' markets in upstate New York as well).

I always imagined farming was hard work. Talking to Deb, hearing just how difficult it is, I'm surprised her beets (deep red ones or plump yellow, almost stripe-y, Chioggia variety) don't cost much more. Though their children used to help in the fields, these days it is just Deb, Pete, and four hired workers. They have 460 CSA members, and nine sites to deliver to. "Everything we do is handwork," she says. The hours are long. Being a CSA farmer means she has to grow fifty different things, so she's also constantly planting new seedlings in the greenhouse, even during growing season when they're harvesting. "Up until July we were still planting and seeding. It's a constant so we have a variety. It's a challenge." Any weeds or bugs they find are removed by hand. "It's not a spray. We are out there. Carrots for us are such an amazing feat. The seeds are so small. They are a thin little whisper of a seed. We direct-seed them. They take two weeks to come up as a tiny, ferny green. Any weed takes that over. To keep and grow carrots, we have to hand-weed them twice. We don't hoe." Watering is also labor intensive. So is handpicking. A tractor does lift and loosen the carrots a bit from the ground, but they pull each bunch out themselves.

The Kavakoses could spray. More and more sprays are becoming allowed under the organic guidelines (especially as more and more corporations get involved with organic standards). But sprays are pricey. "You always have to say, 'Is it going to be worth it?' " If it doesn't work, they're out a lot of money. Instead Deb and Pete rely on giant sheets of row cover, which need to be rolled out, laid down, and sod-stapled to the ground to keep out bugs.

I thought maybe they got a break in the winter, but they don't. CSA season ends in mid-November. In December, they clean up and put equipment away for the next year. January is paperwork month. They order seeds, do their taxes (farm taxes are due in March), and deal with time-consuming and expensive certification issues. Each January they're required to fill out a book of spray records, harvest records, and storage records. They have to have a paper trail for everything they buy and use. Then a certifying inspector comes to the farm and goes through everything, talks to them, and visits the fields

feel you're so regulated, which is almost in opposition to being or-
Come February they're already in the greenhouse in order to have let-
greens in time for their eager members come June.

Pete's daughter recently had her first child. Throughout her pregnancy, she
her parents' farm and from her own garden. "I think the lifestyle you lead goes
the next generation," says Deb. "It's part of everyone's own choice. Supporting local
ional agriculture in any form is going to be healthier for everyone."

This is just a slice of small-farm local organics. Deb can't speak about big-farm methods. But in my mind it carries over. Am I going to spend a little more to help a farmer (and
his or her family) not have to breathe in harmful sprays, treat the earth right (which gives
back to my kids and other people's kids and so on), and get better-tasting, pesticide- and
herbicide-free, nutrient-rich produce? It's a no-brainer. During the growing season, I only
have to think this way about meat and fruit, but come winter I'm making the same decisions as anyone else in that supermarket aisle. I try to choose things grown closest to my
home state and if need be I spend a little extra.

FINDING A CSA NEAR YOU

Local Harvest: *www.localharvest.org*
Using the Local Harvest map, you can find all the farmers' markets, family farms,
locally grown produce, grass-fed livestock, and other sources of sustainably grown
food in your area.

Robyn Van En Center for CSA Resources: *www.csacenter.org*
The center offers a variety of services to existing and new CSA farmers and share-
holders nationally.

FOOD SITES WE LOVE

(With special thanks to Pamela Koch, Nutrition Professor
at Columbia Teachers College)

Vegetable Program UMass Amherst: *www.umassvegetable.org*
This program provides lots of information about farming in the Northeast and more details on CSAs.

Slow Food: *www.slowfood.com*
Founded by Carlo Petrini in Italy in 1986, Slow Food is an international association that promotes food and wine culture and also defends food and agricultural biodiversity worldwide.

Community Food Security Coalition: *www.foodsecurity.org*
A nonprofit organization that believes in building strong, sustainable local, and regional food systems that ensure access to affordable, nutritious, and culturally appropriate food for all people at all times.

Center for Ecoliteracy: *www.ecoliteracy.org*
This center is dedicated to education for sustainable living.

National Campaign for Sustainable Agriculture: *www.sustainableagriculture.net*
This campaign educates the public on the importance of a sustainable food and agricultural system that is economically viable, environmentally sound, socially just, and humane. Get on their action alert list to get involved.

Fair Trade Certified: *www.transfairusa.org/content/support*
When you buy Fair Trade Certified coffee, tea, rice, tropical fruit, or chocolate, you are enabling farmers to live with dignity and invest in their families, their communities, and the environment. Buying fair-trade helps sow the seeds for a better life for producers and their families around the world.

The True Food Network: *www.truefoodnow.org*
This site provides information on genetically engineered foods. Click on "Shopper's Guide" to see and print a list of non-GE products.

Center for Science in the Public Interest: *www.cspinet.org*
Since 1971, this center has been a strong advocate for nutrition and health, food safety, alcohol policy, and sound science.

eating out

You can't always eat at home. While getting the hang of eating organic (it can become addictive), this can create some problems. If you have to eat out, one meal won't harm you or your future baby (yes, there are certain diet restrictions you shouldn't ignore when dining out and pregnant, but more on those in Part 2). There are several ways to go to a restaurant and still keep your organic self satisfied at the same time. Many restaurants now serve local, sustainable, and even organic food. If you're meeting friends for dinner, you might suggest one. If you can't find one to suggest, or if you're subject to someone else's choice, it might be harder to stick to organic. In situations like these, there are always whole foods to fall back on.

Italian menus are pretty easy to navigate, because the cuisine is usually simple and fresh. Less so for French food, which goes heavy on meat and buttery sauces. Chinese can be a great option—brown rice and vegetables, what could be wrong?—as long as you avoid the greasier sauces and fried items. Japanese can also work, especially soup, but the fried dishes and raw fish, once pregnant, should be left alone. Opt for whole-wheat burritos and brown rice when eating Mexican, instead of fried tacos and tortilla chips. Greek and Middle Eastern restaurants have plenty of beans and lentils to choose from, as well as whole-wheat

WHERE TO EAT

- Check out Chefs Collaborative's national network of more than 1,000 members of the food community who promote sustainable cuisine by committing to local, seasonal, and artisanal cooking. Their members' restaurants (in almost all states) are listed at *www.chefscollaborative.org*
- Local Harvest has a solid database of restaurants across America: *www.localharvest.org/restaurants*
- Type in your ZIP code on the Eat Well Guide site for local listings: *www.eatwellguide.org*

rganic pregnancy

pitas and whole-grain salads. When tucking into the breadbasket, choose whole-grain varieties. To avoid hormones, antibiotics, and other unknowns, order low on the food chain—vegetarian options are usually your best bet, especially pasta made with a sauce of some of the safer conventional vegetables (see pages 94–96). Use common sense and enjoy. After all, you're out.

If you're having dinner at a friend's home, eat what is served or quietly avoid what you must. It's important to be a good guest. Don't fret so much about what you would and wouldn't eat if it were up to you. The decision has already been made.

GOOD-BYE TO ALL THAT

Here's a list of what you should gorge on before you have to give it up.

Sushi—Raw meat and fish aren't options for pregnant women.

Oysters—Raw shellfish is a no-no.

Soft cheese—Kiss feta, blue, Brie, and all soft cheeses good-bye. *Listeria* can linger in them even when pasteurized. This is a bacterium your adult system can handle, but it can be life-threatening to a fetus.

Peanuts—Some food allergists believe that eating peanuts and peanut butter when pregnant increases the chance of your baby developing allergies. Other nuts are good substitutes.

Deli sandwiches—Sandwich meat needs to be heated to 165 degrees F to kill any possibly harmful bacteria.

Raw or undercooked eggs—Make sure to cook eggs until the yolks are firm, to avoid risk of salmonella. Also avoid food made with raw eggs like key lime pie, hollandaise sauce, and chocolate mousse.

Rare meat—Underdone meat can contain dangerous bacteria.

Pâté—All types of pâté, even vegetable, can contain *Listeria*.

Refrigerated smoked seafood—This includes lox and whitefish.

My Organic Coming-of-Age

BY LISA M. HAMILTON

It's no secret that I'm a fussy eater. When friends invite me over for dinner, they'll call ahead with the proposed menu so I can tell them what I will and won't eat. When my husband shops for groceries, he does so in fear. He unpacks them cautiously (often after I've left the room), knowing that despite his careful studying, at least one item is likely to break some fine-print rule.

The pickiness began when I was a child, but the first time I made a food choice for reasons other than personal taste, I was thirteen. At a friend's house, I watched *Faces of Death*, a documentary comprised of footage showing real deaths of all kinds. The slaughterhouse scene killed me. The next day, I became a vegetarian.

Before long my conscience began to nag. Why had I forsaken only meat, when *Diet for a New America* and other such books made clear the violence done to dairy cows and laying hens? My high school cafeteria was not so sensitive to such considerations, but the day after graduation my best friend and I crossed cheese, milk, eggs, and all their derivatives off our lists. That first summer yielded a series of disappointing culinary adventures, among them almond milk, soy cheese, and ice cream made from rice. But by my second year of college, I had conquered the challenge of a vegan diet. I cooked nearly all my own meals and had specialties like lasagna with ricotta made from tofu and a chocolate chip cookie recipe based in maple syrup. I even mastered a chocolate cake that, in the absence of eggs, rose from the combination of baking soda and vinegar. Being a vegan had become easy, at least when I stayed home.

Then I met Jim McGinn.

Jim was a farmer of the new, organic variety, who had gone back to school to study literature and environmental science while getting his vegetable farm up and running. When I threw a potluck one February night and served as the centerpiece my tofu-ricotta lasagna, he asked me if I had ever thought about where its tomatoes and red peppers came from in the middle of winter.

I knew Price Chopper was not the answer, so I stayed silent as Jim enlightened me as to why one should not buy warm-weather fruits during cold-weather seasons; why one might choose things theretofore unknown to me—kale, chard, rutabagas—grown locally, rather than buy food imported from Mexico and Chile.

It was solid logic, even if it was tough to swallow. After we talked, my lasagna's bright colors seemed garish against the winter night. While I was not drawn to the dull-looking kale-barley concoction that Jim had contributed, shortly thereafter, I became a local-, organic-, seasonal-eating vegan. My conscience wouldn't have it any other way.

The summers were no problem, my plates filled with the bounty of the vegetable garden and the farmers' market. But then came winter. Without the foresight to grow a winter garden that first year, I found myself living on a diet of nearly all cold-storage carbohydrates—potatoes, carrots, wheat flour. Every meal I ate was some shade of white. By February, I weighed thirty pounds more than I do now and longed for spring just so I could eat some roughage. When Jim's farming partner heard about this in March, he brought me a bag of Swiss chard. I nearly cried with gratitude.

Fast-forward ten years to last winter, to my New Year's Eve dinner party. The meal consisted of a winter salad, artichokes, and a panade, but also short ribs, crab cakes, and homemade chili aioli. Butter was everywhere.

The way I choose my food now is no less intentional—or political—than in college, but I use a different set of considerations. Where my choices used to be a protest of things I opposed, today they are instead votes in favor of the things I believe in.

The shift has come from connecting my food choices to the larger world in which they exist. After studying community development and farming in college, I became a writer who focuses on sustainable agriculture. I believe that organic and other alternative methods of growing food are not simply a matter of giving up pesticides; they are part of a larger movement to reconnect us with the sources of our food and create a bond that transcends mere supermarket shopping.

My real turning point came when I moved to Hawaii, just after college. The local, seasonal, vegan diet was no problem, with papaya and bananas growing outside my window and tomatoes ripe year-round. But during dinner with my boyfriend one evening, I realized that something else had shifted.

I was eating tofu. The soybeans from which it was made had been grown in Iowa, roughly 4,000 miles away, by someone I didn't know. They had been trucked to California, processed by others I didn't know, put in a plastic container, and shipped over 2,300 ocean miles before landing in the local grocery store where I had bought them, then brought them home and seasoned them with another soy concoction of anonymous origins.

My beau was eating an ahi steak. The fish from which it was cut had been caught the day before, by a man who lived down the road from us. He had caught the fish maybe a mile offshore in the ocean visible from our porch, then brought it back, sold it to the man who owned the little fish store on the highway—ten miles from the harbor and four miles from us—who cut it up on the table behind the counter and sold a piece to my boyfriend. Here were two things I believed in deeply, suddenly opposed to each other: I could eat tofu and boycott death, or I could eat ahi and support a local food system. How to make sense of that?

My diet went from being a set of yes-and-no questions to a scale that balanced many issues at once. Ultimately I chose to eat the fish instead of the tofu, but still I did not return to eating meat or dairy products. Then I moved to coastal California, where ahi and bananas are as foreign as tofu is to Hawaii, but green pastures and milk cows are common. Cheese made its way to my plate, as did eggs and the occasional chicken—all from farms that were part of my community. Beef was off the list until years later when I visited Wyoming to interview a rancher named Tony Malmberg. He was boldly striking out on his own, slowly building a market for his organic beef among his neighbors so he could leave the world of international meatpacking conglomerates. I had my first hamburger in fifteen years.

My intention here is not to convert vegetarians to eating local meat. My point is that everything we eat comes with consequences, and eating in a truly conscious way requires one to acknowledge that. Yes, a hamburger means that an animal has died. But dairy cows, in order to produce milk, are continuously impregnated; the resulting calves are either raised for slaughter or they replace other mothers, who go on to become ground beef. Even vegetables and fruit can have a bloody past: According to the Pesticide Action Network, each year 672 million birds are exposed to agricultural pesticides, and an estimated 10 percent (or 67 million) die as a result. Massive accidental pesticide spills from the vegetable and fruit fields of California's Central Valley have killed fish in surrounding rivers even 1 million at a time.

Factor in our food choices' ramifications for the environment, the economy, and people, including farm workers, family farmers, and the meat cutters made famous in *Fast*

Food Nation—not to mention our own fragile bodies and the children that we bear—and it's enough to make you stop eating altogether.

But for me, knowing the facts doesn't act as an appetite suppressant. In fact, buying, cooking, and eating food is the greatest joy in my life. I go to the farmers' market the way others go to church: With each trip I connect to something meaningful and exciting. It's a weekly ritual, where I see old friends and meet new people. I get information and perspectives that change my view of the world, and walk away nearly every time feeling rejuvenated and hopeful. I go there not to boycott the grim, modern food system and its dire consequences, but as a vote in favor of an alternative: namely food that is healthy for the land, the people who grow it, and me.

The diet that results is not an ism, it's a series of considerations. I choose my vegetables and fruits to be grown as close as possible to where I am. Because I live in California, that usually means within seventy-five miles, year-round. When traveling, I apply that standard as well. I seek out restaurants that value sustainable agriculture and track down each new city's farmers' market. When I end up in a truck stop, I still choose potatoes over tomatoes in winter, knowing full well that the choice matters only in principle. (I don't cut corners with animal products, however, eating them only when I know the person who raised the animals and trust his or her methods to be humane.)

But these are my personal priorities. To another person I wouldn't recommend these guidelines so much as the thinking behind them. If you don't like something about the food industry, don't support it. But perhaps more important, do support something you do believe in, so that the alternative can grow. A woman I once interviewed told me that when she was pregnant, she saw herself as eating not just for herself and her baby, but for her grandchildren. The choices we make now not only shield us from the hazards of the present, but they pave the path for a future that's safer for our children.

LISA M. HAMILTON *is a writer and photographer. Her work has been published in* The Nation, Orion, Gastronomica, Utne, *and* National Geographic Traveler.

return to the source

Thirsty? Soon you won't have a ton of choices. Fruit juices in general are pumped full of sugar. Those that aren't—like juice bar juice—are rarely pasteurized and might contain harmful bacteria. This isn't an issue for adults, but pregnant women and children should avoid fresh-squeezed juices. (The FDA agrees.) If you're fresh-squeezing oranges in the morning at home and are meticulously cleaning your juicer, we'd be hard-pressed to tell you to stop. But in general, the main thing you should be getting used to drinking is water. (For more on water filters, see page 38.)

coffee

When you're trying to get pregnant, there are two major liquid habits you might be struggling to give up: alcohol and caffeine. No amount of alcohol has been proven to be safe when pregnant. While caffeine has not been shown to have a negative effect on sperm, some studies maintain that women who drink little or none may take less time to conceive. A study by the *American Journal of Epidemiology* found that people who consumed more than 300 mg of caffeine per day were twice as likely to have conception delayed for a year or more. When it came to us, we decided to give up both. It wasn't easy. It was particularly difficult during the preconception phase, as there was less incentive to go without. Once morning sickness hit, it wasn't as hard.

If you're drinking coffee, try whenever possible to buy fair-trade, shade-grown, and/or organic. Fair trade, according to the certifying agency TransFair USA, helps family farmers in developing countries gain direct access to international markets and allows them to receive fair prices for their products. Shade-grown coffee is just that—grown on shaded, forestlike land as opposed to on plantations that have been cleared of trees. Coffee grown in the direct sunlight provides no habitat for migratory birds and requires more pesticides and fertilizers.

tea

Tea is becoming a bit like wine these days; connoisseurs are into harvest dates, and whole leaves from specific regions. The upside is that stores like In Pursuit of Tea (*www.inpursuitoftea.com*) and tea rooms like Samovar Tea Lounge (*www.samovartea.com*) are sprouting up everywhere to sell and serve well-produced tea, much of which is organic. Even if the producers haven't gone to the extra expense to get organically certified, the tea is often chemical-free. The person you're buying from should be able to answer any questions you have. The extra flavors in whole-leaf or boxed tea like Earl Grey tend to be synthetic, so be sure to ask about that. When brewing tea, use filtered water.

decaf, anyone?

If you're buying decaf, look for water-processed versions; chemical processing leaves behind chemicals you don't want in your system. Decaf also contains a small amount of caffeine. The only things that are truly caffeine-free are herbals (not technically tea). If you can't find water-processed decaf tea, try this trick: Steep a low-in-caffeine tea (like green or white) for twenty to forty seconds. Pour out the liquid. Then resteep. This gets rid of about 80 percent of the caffeine, but a quality tea will retain much of the flavor.

the sipping news

If you find you're not pregnant this month, choose organic wine to drink during the two-week window until you try again. Grapes are generally sprayed heavily with pesticides. Since wine is made from fermented grapes, it makes sense to try to buy wines from unsprayed grapes. Until recently, organic wine was considered tasteless and not worthy of regard by wine snobs. Part of the reason organic wine doesn't always taste great is that it doesn't contain added sulfites, which act as a preservative. Luckily these days you can buy wine made with organic grapes and added sulfur dioxide, which makes for nearly organic (and delicious) wine. Though these wines can't be officially labeled as organic, you will often find "made with organically grown grapes" or something similar stamped on the bottle. There are also a growing number of high-quality biodynamic wines now available. The biodynamic farming method is said to integrate organic agriculture, the role of farm animals, and the rhythm and cycles of the earth, moon, and stars. Seriously. So far most of these wines come from France. Stateside, three big names making wine with organic grapes are Bonterra, Frey, and Sinskey.

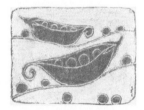

CHAPTER TWO

home environment

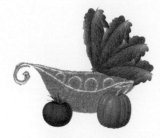

If you're like us, there's a chance you didn't pay that much attention to the noxious poisons lurking under the kitchen sink and around the house until you started seriously thinking about getting pregnant. You're going to clean up your body for your new houseguest, so it makes sense to do the same to your actual house, especially since once she's born, your baby will spend about 90 percent of her early life indoors.

The amount of information to consider in the following pages might overwhelm you. Don't let it. First we'll discuss some of the effects of household toxins. Then we'll zero in on what you can control.

defensive living

When it comes to your unborn child, it's smart to be suspicious and start living a little more defensively. Since World War II, at least 75,000 new synthetic chemical compounds have been developed and released into the environment. (To find out how toxic your hometown is, go to *Scorecard.org* and type in your ZIP code. Very satisfying—if you happen to live in Marin County, California.) In her amazing book *Living Downstream*, ecologist, author, and cancer survivor Sandra Steingraber offers a wealth of evidence linking cancer and environmental contamination.

- One-half of the world's cancers occur among people in industrialized countries, even though industrialized countries account for only one-fifth of the population.
- Breast cancer rates are thirty times higher in the United States than in parts of Africa.
- The International Agency for Research on Cancer has concluded that 80 percent of all cancer is attributable to environmental influences (including smoking and exposure to carcinogenic chemicals).
- During our lifetime, 40 percent of all Americans will get some form of cancer—50 percent of men, 30 percent of women.

cleaning

Today's cleaning products are made from a shocking number of toxic chemicals. When used, the chemicals in them can stay suspended in the air for hours and even days for easy inhalation. This explains the red eyes and headache that follow a good cleaning, and the way the skin on your fingers feels shredded after scrubbing the tub with bleach. Dangerous chemicals also stick around on surfaces and can be absorbed when skin comes into contact with them. Possibly most disturbing is the fact that when different cleaners accidentally come into contact with each other, they can create entirely new toxic substances.

Pre-pregnancy is the perfect time to get under your sink and evaluate all the cleaning products you've acquired over the years. Don't stop at bathroom and living room cleaners; dishwasher and laundry detergents can be just as bad. You'll want to get rid of everything that isn't completely nontoxic. Either give them to someone who isn't trying to get pregnant, or use them up quickly and replace them with something nontoxic. For the greenest products available for every cleaning job you can imagine, see *The Green Guide*'s Household Cleaning and Laundry product reports and Smart Shopper's wallet-size cards at *www.thegreenguide.com*. (A $15 year-long subscription includes access to extra valuable content and was a big help to us while we were transitioning.)

The Environmental Protection Agency (EPA) has found the air quality in our homes to be two to five times more toxic than the air outside—contaminated by somewhere between 20 and 150 different pollutants (*www.epa.gov*). A lot of this pollution comes from petrochemical cleaners (made from petroleum or gas). One of the main reasons we aren't as suspicious of cleaning products as we should be is that labels on cleaning products aren't required to warn us about their hazardous ingredients. Ingredients are considered "trade secrets" and are protected by government regulations. A study by a New York City Poison Control Center found that 85 percent of product warning labels are inadequate. It's anybody's guess what's really in your cleaning products, which is part of the reason New York Governor George Pataki passed a bill requiring the use of green cleaning solutions in schools statewide as of September 2006.

There are plenty of nontoxic alternatives on the market from brands like Ecover and Seventh Generation, but the fact is that some mixture of borax, vegetable-based liquid soap, water, club soda, white vinegar, baking soda, and lemon will take care of pretty much anything you want to clean. If you don't have the time or energy to find a home brew that works for you, do what we did and reduce your cleaning arsenal to three affordable and nontoxic items: liquid soap, white vinegar, and baking soda. For cleaning glass, mix equal parts vinegar and water. For jobs that require some grit, mix liquid soap and baking soda into a paste. For everything else, liquid soap and water will do the trick. For other home remedy recipes check out two of our most dog-eared resources, *Home Safe Home* by Debra Lynn Dadd and *Better Basics for the Home* by Annie Berthold-Bond.

THE HAZARDS OF HOUSEHOLD CLEANERS
(THE COMPANIES THAT MAKE YOUR CLEANING PRODUCTS AREN'T REQUIRED TO LIST THEIR INGREDIENTS BECAUSE THEY ARE CONSIDERED TRADE SECRETS)

Alkyl Phenoxy Polyethoxy Ethanols
FOUND IN: Conventional laundry detergents, all-purpose cleaners, and hard-surface cleaners
Also known as nonyl phenoxy ethoxylate or nonyl phenol ethoxylate. Researchers in England have found that in trace amounts these synthetic surfactants activate estrogen receptors in cells, which in turn alters the activity of certain genes. For example, in experiments they have been found to stimulate the growth of breast cancer cells and feminize male fish.

Ammonia
FOUND IN: Glass cleaners, all-purpose cleaners, and disinfectants
An irritant that affects the skin, eyes, and respiratory passages. Heavy exposure can cause bronchial damage, chemical burns, cataracts, and corneal damage.

Amyl Acetate

FOUND IN: Conventional furniture polishes

This synthetic grease cutter is a neurotoxin implicated in central nervous system depression.

Aromatic Hydrocarbons

FOUND IN: Conventional heavy-duty degreasers and deodorizers

These synthetic compounds are members of the benzene family of chemicals. Though not all are carcinogenic, they're hazardous. They also contaminate air and groundwater.

Benzene

(also benzol, benzole, annulene, benzeen, phenyl hydride, coal naphtha)

FOUND IN: Conventional oven cleaners, detergents, furniture polish, and spot removers

Made from petroleum and coal, benzene is classified by the International Agency for Research on Cancer as a carcinogen. It's listed in the 1990 Clean Air Act as a hazardous air pollutant, and is on the EPA's Community Right-to-Know list. It's not something you want to add to the air you're breathing at home.

Butyl Cellosolve

(also butoxyethanol, butyl oxitol, ethylene glycol monobutyl ether, hydroxypropyl methylcellulose)

FOUND IN: Conventional spray cleaners, all-purpose cleaners, and abrasive cleaners

This toxic synthetic solvent and grease cutter can irritate mucous membranes and cause liver and kidney damage. Butyl cellosolve is also a neurotoxin that can depress the nervous system and cause a variety of associated problems.

Chlorine

(also hypochlorite, sodium hypochlorite, sodium dichloroisocyanurate, hydrogen chloride, hydrochloric acid)

FOUND IN: Conventional laundry bleach, dishwasher detergent, scouring powders, and basin, tub, and tile cleaners

Chlorine, the chemical most frequently involved in household poisonings in the United States, is listed in the 1990 Clean Air Act as a hazardous air pollutant and is on the EPA's Community Right-to-Know list. In 1993, the American Public Health Association issued a resolution calling for the gradual phase-out of most organochlorine compounds. First manufactured on an industrial scale in the early 1900s, it was used as a poison in World War I. In addition to its direct toxic effects on living organisms, chlorine also reacts with materials in the environment to create other hazardous and carcinogenic toxins, including trihalomethanes (THMs), chloroform, and organochlorines, an extremely dangerous class of compounds that cause reproductive, endocrine, and immune system disorders. The most well known organochlorine is dioxin. Products containing chlorine (or any of its derivatives or precursors) should be avoided at all costs. Similarly, any chemical with "-chlor-" as part of its name, or any ingredient listed as "bleach" should be considered unacceptable.

Crystalline Silica

FOUND IN: All-purpose cleaners, bathroom cleaners, and abrasive cleaners

This carcinogen acts as an eye, skin, and lung irritant.

Dioxane

(also diethylene dioxide, diethylene ether, diethylene oxide)

FOUND IN: Conventional window cleaners

The EPA classified this solvent as a probable human carcinogen, and some research suggests that it may suppress the immune system. Dioxane is listed in the 1990 Clean Air Act as a hazardous air pollutant and is on the EPA's Community Right-to-Know list.

Ethyl Alcohol

FOUND IN: Detergents, disinfectants, carpet cleaners, tub and tile cleaners, and air fresheners

This mild eye, skin, and respiratory tract irritant can be absorbed by inhalation and across the skin. It's also a central nervous system depressant.

Ethyl Cellosolve

FOUND IN: Conventional all-purpose cleaners and window cleaners

A synthetic solvent, ethyl cellosolve is both a nasal irritant and a neurotoxin.

Ethylene Glycol

(also ethylene dihydrate, ethylene alcohol)

FOUND IN: Conventional all-purpose cleaners

The vapors of this highly toxic synthetic solvent (it's a nasal irritant and a neurotoxin) contribute to the formation of urban ozone pollution. Ethylene glycol is listed in the 1990 Clean Air Act as a hazardous air pollutant and is on the EPA's Community Right-to-Know list.

Formaldehyde

FOUND IN: Conventional deodorizers, disinfectants, germicides, adhesives, permanent press fabrics, and particleboard

Although uncommon as a primary ingredient, formaldehyde is present as a contaminant in many consumer household products. It has been shown to cause cancer in animals, may cause it in humans, and is a respiratory irritant. Products containing formaldehyde, which may appear as a preservative, should be avoided. It can cause watery eyes, burning sensations in the eyes and throat, nausea, and difficulty in breathing in some people, especially when exposed at elevated levels. High concentrations may also trigger attacks in people with asthma.

Hydrochloric Acid

(also chlorine and muriatic acid)

FOUND IN: Conventional toilet bowl cleaners and deodorizers

This strong mineral is a severe eye, skin, and mucous membrane irritant, and is highly toxic if inhaled. Inhalation of vapors may cause severe irritation of the respiratory system, coughing, and difficulty breathing. Its systemic effects are unknown.

Hydroxyacetic Acid

FOUND IN: Dishwasher detergents and hard-surface cleaners

This acid is used to help adjust pH in products. It may be a liver and kidney toxicant.

Kerosene

FOUND IN: Conventional all-purpose cleaners and abrasives, furniture polishes, and degreasers

A synthetic distillate used as a grease cutter, kerosene can damage lung tissues and dissolve the fatty tissue that surrounds nerve cells.

Methanol

FOUND IN: Conventional glass cleaners

This acutely toxic solvent derived from wood, natural gas, or petroleum can cause blindness.

Organic Solvents

FOUND IN: Conventional all-purpose cleaners, degreasers, and metal polishes

This category of solvents and grease-cutters are mostly of synthetic origin (organic in this instance refers to their petroleum origins. Organic solvents are generally neurotoxins and nervous system depressants, especially in large quantities.

Paradichlorobenzene

(also p-Dichlorobenzene, PDCB)

FOUND IN: Mothballs and deodorizers

PDCB is a chlorinated synthetic of extreme chronic toxicity and environmental concern. Paradichlorobenzene is an endocrine disrupter and carcinogen. In other words, mothballs are not an option.

Phosphoric Acid

FOUND IN: Conventional bathroom cleaners

A toxic chemical on the EPA's Community Right-to-Know list, phosphoric acid is also controlled under the Clean Air Act as an air pollutant. The Occupational Safety and Health Administration (OSHA) regulates the maximum allowable levels in the workplace to protect workers.

Quaternium 15

FOUND IN: Conventional detergents, deodorizers, and disinfectants

What you need to know about this alkyl ammonium is that it releases formaldehyde, a potent toxin.

Sodium Hydroxide

FOUND IN: Conventional oven cleaners and drain cleaners

Think twice before pouring this stuff down your drain or spraying in your oven. It's a strong, caustic substance that causes severe corrosive damage to eyes, skin, and mucous membranes, as well as the mouth, throat, esophagus, and stomach. Blindness is reported in animals exposed to as little as 2% dilution for just one minute. Skin is typically damaged by 0.12% dilutions for a period of one hour. Tests with healthy volunteers exposed to the chemical in spray from oven cleaners showed that respiratory tract irritation developed in two to fifteen minutes. Sodium hydroxide is included as a toxic chemical on the EPA's Community Right-to-Know list. It is also a controlled substance in the workplace, and OSHA has set limitations on concentrations in the air.

Trisodium Nitrilotriacetate (NTA)

FOUND IN: Conventional stain removers, laundry detergents, carpet treatments, and dishwasher detergents

This suspected human carcinogen, a synthetic amino-polycarboxylic acid chelating agent, is listed as such by California's Proposition 65, Workers' Right-to-Know legislation. It also impedes the elimination of heavy metals in wastewater treatment, creating an environmental hazard.

THE TOP TEN CHEMICALS MOST LIKELY
TO BE FOUND IN YOUR HOME

1. Nonylphenol ethoxylates: economy laundry detergents, all-purpose spray cleaners
2. 2-Butoxyethanol (butyl cellosolve, ethylene glycol monobutyl ether): all-purpose spray cleaners, glass cleaners
3. Chlorine bleach (sodium hypochlorite): automatic dishwasher detergents, kitchen and bathroom cleaners, laundry detergent
4. Triclosan: antimicrobial cleaners
5. Phthalates: plastics—especially polyvinyl chloride (PVC), air fresheners
6. Polybrominated diphenyl ethers (PBDEs): computer cases, foam pads
7. Formaldehyde: particleboard furniture and doors, air fresheners, floor and furniture waxes
8. Cigarette smoke (nitrogen oxides, hydrogen cyanide, carbon monoxide, nicotine, tar, formaldehyde, ammonia, and arsenic)
9. Polyvinyl chloride (PVC): clear, flexible plastics (photo album sheets), flexible molded toys
10. Paradichlorobenzene (p-Dichlorobenzene): mothballs

house detox

Once you've overhauled your cleaning products, the next thing you want to do is find out how healthy your home is. This means thinking about slightly harder-to-manage issues like lead paint, mold, vinyl, and pressed wood. If you can afford to, get a professional environmental assessment. Otherwise, we'll guide you through the potential hazards. The most important piece of advice we have to give you is that if you plan to do any renovations, *do them now, before you get pregnant*. Over half of pregnancies are unplanned, so if you find you're already pregnant, you should remove yourself for the overhaul or just skip the renovation entirely so that you aren't exposed to threatening chemicals. We realize that you might not want to build a nursery before you even begin trying, so we're saving our nontoxic nursery guide for Part 2. But if you want to designate a room for the baby and need to build or tear down any walls, now's the time to do it. What follows is a short glossary of hidden household toxins that you may not yet be aware of, but that we'll be referring to in the pages to come.

PCBs Polychlorinated biphenyls are a group of toxic chemicals used for a variety of purposes and found in a number of products, such as carbonless copy paper, adhesives, hydraulic fluids, and caulking compounds. They were originally used to insulate electrical equipment, and although they've been banned in the United States since the late seventies, they are still found in water. They accumulate in the sediment at the bottoms of rivers and lakes, and build up in the fatty tissues of fish. The primary effect of PCBs is on the endocrine system, which is responsible for regulating the hormones in our bodies. They are particularly dangerous to fetuses and young children. If PCBs get into your bloodstream, they can upset the body's natural hormone levels and can lead to birth defects and cancers.

PBDEs Considered the new PCBs, polybrominated diphenyl ethers are a group of brominated flame retardants used in lots of products, including the foam in couches and mattresses, and plastic TV and computer monitors (Dell and HP, among others, have banned them). One of the reasons PBDEs are so hard to avoid is that they're not bound to the molecules in materials, so toxic residue can escape in the form of dust. Most kinds of PBDEs have been banned in Europe since 2004, and American women carry ten to seventy times as many PBDEs in their breast milk, tissues, and blood as Europeans do. Exposure to PBDEs during fetal development can negatively affect how the brain functions.

VOCs Volatile organic compounds are chemicals that easily form vapors at normal temperature. The term usually describes solvents, certain paint additives, aerosols, fuels (such as gasoline and kerosene), dry-cleaning solutions, and a variety of other products ranging from office supplies to building materials.

PVC Polyvinyl chloride is one of the most widely used and environmentally hazardous plastics produced. PVC is a hard plastic that is made softer and more flexible by the addition of phthalates (see below). PVC is used in vinyl siding, records, pipe/plumbing/conduit fixtures, and, in its soft form, for clothing, upholstery, bean bag chairs, and car seats. Vinyl chloride is a known human carcinogen that can lead to a number of cancers, endocrine disruption, endometriosis, neurological damage, birth defects, impaired child development, and reproductive and immune system damage. PVC releases dioxins during its manufacture and disposal and cannot be easily recycled because of its chlorine and additive content. Many companies (including Microsoft and Kaiser Permanente) are phasing out PVC plastic in their products and packaging.

Phthalates are a family of chemicals used in many beauty products and to give flexibility to PVC in everything from the kitchen floor to your baby's bib. They can cause an array of health problems, including heart, lung, and blood pressure problems and kidney and liver failure, but the most troubling is their effect on the reproductive development of fetuses, particularly males. In September 2004, the European Union banned the use of some phthalate plasticizers in children's toys, including those that kids under three would be prone to put in their mouths. There are also lots of phthalates in beauty products (see page 78). Unfortunately, phthalates are still allowed in the United States, but many companies are voluntarily making PVC-free toys.

> **Formaldehyde** is a preservative commonly found in cosmetics, glue (including glue [that]
> materials together, like plywood and particleboard), and paint, and is a probable c[arcinogen]
> National Toxicology Program.

> **PFOA or C8** (perfluorooctanoic acid) is a toxic chemical used in making food wr[ap]
> coatings, and nonstick pan coatings like Teflon. PFOA exposure during pregnan[cy]
> weight in mice, and many of the exposed offspring went on to experience de[velopmental]
> admitted that it may be unsafe to humans and the environment. DuPont, th[e]
> States, and several major producers worldwide have agreed to phase out the chemical un[der]
> program.

lead

It's been banned for use in paint since 1978, but lead (a naturally occurring heavy metal) still shows up in gasoline, PVC plastic, pipes, ceramic glazes, caulk, and old paint. These days it's also used in the production of batteries, ammunition, metal products (solder and pipes), devices to shield X-rays, and computer monitors (to block radiation). It's added to certain kinds of plastic, such as vinyl blinds, as well as the ink on plastic grocery bags. Developing babies can be exposed to lead in the womb.

The EPA says more than 80 percent of U.S. homes built before 1978 (about 64 million) still contain some amount of lead. If your home was built before then, test it! All home buyers and tenants have the legal right to be informed of the presence of lead paint in pre-1987 homes they're buying or renting. The National Lead Information Center (NLIC) provides a list of EPA-certified labs near you where you can send paint chips from cracks to be tested. They'll also give you a list of local specialists who can either remove or seal the lead. Do-it-yourself spot test kits will give you a quick idea of whether you have lead in paint chips, but they are not approved by the EPA or the U.S. Department of Housing and Urban Development (HUD) because they give only a yes-no type answer, not a quantitative lab result (a number that can be compared with the federal standards).

If lead is found, but the paint is still intact (not chipping or peeling), then you're basically safe. However, if the lead paint is falling apart or was used on doorjambs or window frames, where constant friction causes dust to escape,

You'll need to take some action. You should never, ever try to get ride of lead paint yourself, especially if pregnant or planning to be. It is too dangerous. You must absolutely hire a lead abatement professional.

To find a contractor in your area, call HUD's Lead Listing's office at 800-424-LEAD or visit *www.leadlisting.com*. Your family should temporarily move until the lead paint is removed.

Many imported and antique ceramics contain some lead. Have them tested, too. And avoid drinking from (or storing food in) leaded crystal.

tap water

There are so many baby-unfriendly pollutants that could be lingering in your water and your pipes that having it tested and filtering it is a must. You can find out where your water can be tested here: *www.epa.gov/safewater/privatewells/labs*, or here: *www.leadtesting.com*. If the results come back with higher than the EPA's limit of .015 mg of lead per liter of household water, you might consider getting a reverse-osmosis system or a distiller. A simple temporary solution is a carbon carafe filter pitcher like Brita or Pur.

types of filters

- Most faucet units and pitchers use carbon filters that absorb lead, chlorine by-products, and some organic chemicals, as well as odors and tastes. They won't remove heavy metals, pesticides, nitrites, bacteria, or microbes, but they are the least-expensive filter type and are sufficient for most needs.
- Ceramic filters, which are often combined with carbon filters, remove bacteria, asbestos, and sediment.
- Distillers boil water into steam, then condense it back into water in a chamber, leaving behind particles and dissolved solids. Since is heated, distillers kill microbes as well as eliminate other ts, including arsenic, but not volatile organic compounds and e, which are usually removed by an accompanying carbon filter.

anic pregnancy

- Installed in showerheads, copper/zinc alloy systems remove chlorine, chloroform, and heavy metals and reduce the contaminants that can be inhaled and absorbed through the skin in water and steam. Just make sure before you buy a system that it doesn't force water to travel up before it goes down through the filter. It makes for impossibly low water pressure. We learned this the hard way.

What Do I Tell My Grandchildren?

BY THEO COLBORN

About ten years ago when people were told there were 70,000 man-made chemicals in use globally, they reared back in their seats in amazement. Five years ago that number jumped to 87,000, and today the figure is over 100,000. Of those 100,000, 5,200 are produced in quantities of over 2 million pounds a year, and one chemical was produced in quantities of over 1.2 billion pounds in one year in the United States alone. Not one of these 100,000 chemicals was thoroughly tested for what it might do to a baby before it is born.

I have to keep reminding myself that because of some of these high-volume chemicals, it has been possible for me to talk to my grandchildren over the phone and send them e-mails when they are over 1,000 miles away. When their home was remodeled recently, many of these chemicals were used in the wood on the floors, the paint on the walls, and in the new energy-saving windows and kitchen appliances that made their home airtight and attractive. The chemicals are also in the computers and monitors, TVs, and other electrical appliances throughout their home; in the soft mattresses and cuddly pillows they sleep and play on; in the clothes they wear; and in almost every one of their personal care products like shampoos, conditioners, soaps, and lotions. Invisible fragments of these chemicals end up in the air, on furniture surfaces, and on the floor where they often play. Coming from the wear and tear of construction materials and warming-up of computers and monitors and other electrical appliances, they become part of what the family inhales and touches every day.

The amount of chemicals in my grandchildren's food may be minor compared with what they are inhaling and absorbing through their skin twenty-four hours a day. In the womb, these chemicals raise havoc during development, disrupting the normal chemical medley that controls how babies develop and how they think and behave later in life. They also interfere with the development of the babies' organs and physiological systems, leading to childhood disorders or, later in life, to infertility or adult-onset disorders and cancers. But do I want to talk about all this to these little tots who are just learning to process information, learning to read, developing some social skills, and at an age when they need to feel secure and loved?

I recently had the exceptional experience of spending some time with my grandchildren on a nearby mountain where we were snowbound most of the time. I watched the younger tots chew and suck on plastic straws that had been filled with honey and a weird-looking thing they called a doll made of a very malleable plastic. For a while I was disturbed that my son and his wife let them do this. They certainly have heard me talk about the "nasties" in plastics for years. How could they allow their children, my grandchildren, to do this? I came away from our mountain retreat feeling blue, frustrated, and upset with myself because I had not been able to convince my own children of the hazards their children, my grandchildren, face every day in our high-tech modern society. But then I remembered that while on our weekend retreat, we ate our meals off plastic-coated disposable plates and occasionally used plastic "silverware," and all the fishing and camping gear we hauled along with us was made of plastic or impregnated with some of these chemicals.

It's tough enough to be a grandmother and not tell my children how to raise their children. But it is even tougher knowing what I do about the stealth health effects of the chemicals upon which society has become dependent. Like addicts, without these chemicals, our society would soon collapse. Yet, I know that some of these chemicals have made products tougher than steel, lighter and stronger than any natural product available, relatively cheap, flameproof, and in the case of lubricants, frictionless—they have made it possible for millions of people to have comfortable and affordable homes, to travel anywhere in the world on a whim.

In retrospection I realized that I am as guilty as my children. Recently, I bought a new car made almost entirely of plastic because I wanted a car that would not use much gasoline. Every time I get in my "wheels," I have to push to the back of my mind that I am exposing myself to chemicals that are not safe. There are still times when I wrap my leftover food in plastic film, carry my water in a plastic bottle, and purchase and use products I know have these dangerous chemicals in them because I need them—and have no choice.

We used to tell our children fairy tales to prepare them for the bad things they might encounter later in life. I have told myself for years that it is time to write some modern-day fairy tales about the more troublesome synthetic chemicals that have become an integral part of our lifestyle. Perhaps more important, because we need to reach children who can't read (because of prenatal exposure to certain chemicals?) or because their parents do not read to them, the time has come for some colorful animated cartoons to play the role of these stealth chemicals that are stealing our children's potential. The trouble is that it is difficult translating science into language that people want to listen to. How often I have wished that Walt Disney were still alive and could tackle the problem. But then again, Disney would never produce a film on this topic—too much of the technology that made it possible for him to share his unique artistic gift with the world is dependent upon the chemicals we now know are eating away at the integrity of each new generation. Even if Disney did produce a cinematographic masterpiece that told the story, corporate pressure would never allow its release. You can bet that those who produce and use the chemicals in their products will continue to assure you that chemical disruption is a preposterous fairy tale. Well, perhaps it is! Just like Humpty Dumpty—for those who have been sabotaged by chemicals before they were born, all of the medical doctors and all of the medical cures cannot put the poor children's brains and organs back together again.

Dr. Theo Colborn is a scientist and one of the world's leading experts on endocrine disrupters. Her work has prompted the enactment of new laws around the world (including Senate Bill S 1391: "Child, Worker, and Consumer-Safe Chemicals Act of 2005") and redirected the research of government and academia. She's a professor of zoology at the University of Florida, Gainesville, and the coauthor of Our Stolen Future.

vinyl

PVC is frequently used in flooring, countertops, mini-blinds, water pipes, and window frames. Unlike a lot of products that you can off-gas by airing out until the fumes are gone, PVC remains toxic. We strongly urge you to use nontoxic or secondhand materials when getting anything "new" for your home (make sure any hand-me-down furniture is made of natural materials, too). This applies to something as small as a vinyl shower curtain and as big as a new car. The manufacture and incineration of PVC creates dioxins, known human carcinogens also linked to reproductive and immune disorders.

radon

Throw open your windows to help reduce radon, an invisible natural radioactive gas (the result of decaying radioactive materials in rocks, soil, minerals, natural gas, and water). Soil and building materials are the biggest sources of radon at home. It's usually produced under the house or in the basement before seeping up through porous cracks to become a dangerous contaminant. It's known to cause lung cancer in high concentrations, but its health effects at lower levels of exposure are unsubstantiated. Still, it's not a risk we'd want to take. The only way to know for sure if you have radon is to get your home tested, which you can do by ordering a test kit from any number of companies, including *www.radonzone.com*, *www.radon.info*, *www.radonmonitor.com*, and *www.gasniffer.com*. All that is usually required to take care of radon is a little more ventilation.

carbon monoxide

Carbon monoxide is a clear, tasteless, odorless gas that is produced from incomplete combustion. Exposure to carbon monoxide can cause headaches; fatigue; dizziness; nausea; permanent damage to the brain, central nervous system, and heart; and even death by reducing the amount of oxygen red blood cells carry. Infants, children, pregnant women, the elderly, and people with heart or respiratory problems are most susceptible to carbon monoxide poisoning. Because you can't see, smell, or taste carbon monoxide, it has to be tested for with a monitor or an alarm, which are now legally required in many states.

mold

We love it on cheese, but twenty-five million Americans have allergic reactions to mold every year. There are varying degrees of exposure. While the term "toxic mold" implies that mold is toxic, it actually refers to something that mold produces called mycotoxin, and reports of mycotoxin found in homes are very uncommon. Allergic reactions to nontoxic mold include nosebleeds, anemia, shortness of breath, wheezing, asthma, skin irritation, rashes, and upper respiratory infections. Infants exposed to high levels of mold at home could also have an increased risk of lower respiratory illnesses such as croup, pneumonia, bronchitis, and bronchiolitis. Mold is found in all of the places you might imagine: where there's moisture, air, and something for the fungus to eat—damp basements, bathrooms, mattresses, plants, and pillows. We advise having the air in your

BUG OFF

There are whole books written on natural pest control, but we personally haven't had much luck getting rid of ants, mice, and cockroaches with suggestions of basil, cayenne, soapy trails, and citrus vinaigrettes. The problem with less-than-natural insecticides is that they contain organophosphates that interfere with the nervous system, which you really don't want to breathe if there is a possibility you might be pregnant. While we have had some luck getting rid of pests with boric acid baits and traps with pheromones (released by roaches to attract other roaches), our main advice is to be more vigilant than you might usually be during an infestation. Also be sure to stuff every hole and entryway you can find in the floors and walls, and to use a nontoxic caulk to seal cracks.

Unfortunately bedbugs are on the rise, and they're maddeningly hard to get rid of. As with mice, ants, and cockroaches, we recommend stuffing every hole, crack, and open seam you can find in your walls and floorboards. They can take up residence in anything from your favorite comforter to your mattress, and if they're still around after you vacuum and clean, you really have only two choices—throw out whatever they've made home (chair, couch, rug), or hermetically seal the bugged item for at least one year in an airtight container.

home tested for mold if you have reason to be suspicious, even if it is pricey. It's possible to have mold that isn't visible, particularly if you've had water damage or have an old roof.

The remainder of this chapter focuses less on hidden dangers in your house and more on specific choices you can make. Next: the safest carpets, furniture, flooring, and paint.

carpet

Wall-to-wall carpets may feel clean, but in reality they're anything but. Usually made of synthetic materials that off-gas, a lot of time they're covered in chemical stain-resistants and backed with chemical adhesives to help bind them together. Most also require glue to adhere them to the floor, which contains VOCs. Whenever possible, we recommend a natural wood floor with a natural fiber throw carpet or rug that can be either tossed in the washing machine or cleaned with a nontoxic carpet shampoo.

DUST MITES

Dust mites are something that will haunt you when you have a baby who spends most of her time on the floor. They're a major source of allergies and asthma attacks, but you can start taking preventative measures now to keep them from thriving. As many as 500 mites can live in a gram of dust, feeding off dead human skin, and the protein in their feces triggers allergies and asthma. These microscopic pests love wall-to-wall carpeting, especially with a thick pile, and thrive in humid, warm environments. They also gather in mattresses, bedding, upholstered furniture, and stuffed animals. You can kill them by washing the sheets every two weeks and cleaning more often, but they are hard to get rid of in wall-to-wall carpeting. If you have to get a carpet, find one made of natural fibers and preferably one that can be washed frequently.

furniture

By this point in your life you've probably spent years collecting pieces of furniture that you like and are hardly prepared to throw them all out because they're made of the wrong materials. We're not suggesting you do. If you're thinking about replacing an expensive item like a living room couch because you're worried about PBDEs in the foam cushions, our advice is don't. In fact, *The Green Guide* editor, Mindy Pennybacker, says that when she couldn't afford an organic cotton couch, she covered hers with a thick layer of natural cotton instead. "I don't think people should obsess about PBDEs to the point where they replace all their furniture at once," says Pennybacker. "Better to block chemicals by putting a wool or cotton pad on the mattress your face is pressed up against every day, regularly wipe up dust where PBDEs collect, and replace crumbling foam

SOURCES FOR SAFER FURNITURE

IKEA: *www.ikea.com* Despite being the juggernaut it is, IKEA supports the use of environmentally friendly, sustainable, and recycled materials and has an environmental policy that doesn't allow the use of PVC, formaldehyde-based glues, brominated flame retardants, or other toxins.
Green Home Environmental: *www.greenhome.com*
White Lotus: *whitelotus.net*
C. G. Sparks: *www.furniturewithsoul .com*
Eco Choices: *www.ecochoices.com*
Furnature: *www.furnature.com*
Q Collection: *www.qcollection.com*
Old Adirondack: *www.oldadirondack .com*
Vivavi: *www.vivavi.com*

ALTERNATIVES TO DANGEROUS BUILDING MATERIALS

(Thanks to the Children's Health Environmental Coalition: *www.checnet .org*).

Agriboard: *www.agriboard.com*
Environmental Home Center: *www .environmentalhomecenter.com*
Finland Color Plywood Corp.: *www .fincolorply.com*
Homasote Co.: *www.homasote.com*
Primeboard: *www.primeboard.com*
The Plastic Lumber Company: *www.plasticlumber.com*
Treated Wood: *www.chemspec.com*

cushions." If you're in the market for something new, there are a number of affordable eco-friendly options from places like IKEA and Environmental Home Center. With a little research, you don't have to remortgage your house for greener furniture.

We suggest avoiding anything made of particleboard or other composites, because the glues that hold them together can give off enough formaldehyde to be dangerous to a growing fetus. Keep in mind that something that looks like a natural piece of wood can have unfinished edges. Plywood and particleboard can be easily hidden behind natural veneers to save the manufacturer money. You also want to avoid furniture that has been treated with stain- and water-resistant finishes, which may release the industrial chemical perfluorooctanoic acid (PFOA). Pick natural materials over plastic, and when building something new, it's also important to buy untreated, natural woods and treat them with nontoxic sealants (see page 115). Check out the Product Reports section of *The Green Guide* (*www .thegreenguide.com*) for current, in-depth reporting on the safest green choices available.

flooring

The safest types of floors are untreated hardwood, true linoleum (the natural material, not the vinyl imitation), ceramic tile, marble, and stone slate. Cork is becoming more popular because it's warmer than tiles and, like linoleum, resilient—a forgiving surface for rolling, tumbling babies and toddlers. Brick, marble, and other stone tiles are more costly but also good choices. The following stores will have what you need.

- Environmental Depot: *www.environproducts.com*
- Conklin's Authentic Barnwood: *www.conklinsbarnwood.com*
- Crossroads Recycled Lumber: *www.crossroadslumber.com*
- Eco Timber International: *www.ecotimber.com*

treating hardwood floors

When staining and/or sealing a hardwood floor, choose water-based instead of solvent-based products. They can be found in most building stores or ordered specifically at the Environmental Home Center (*www.environmentalhomecenter.com*). Natural finishes such as tung oil look beautiful and can be coated with beeswax, which needs to be reapplied only around once a year.

fireplaces

Everyone loves the warm glow of a fireplace, but when you think of the headache and watery eyes that often accompany the experience, it makes sense that they're not completely safe—particularly for pregnant women. Among other things, the smoke produced by burning wood can contain carbon monoxide, formaldehyde, and tiny smoke particles that sometimes have toxic compounds attached. Breathing wood smoke can also reduce lung function and exacerbate allergies and existing diseases like asthma. The greatest health risk, as usual, is to fetuses, infants, and children.

paint

One of our basic rules of thumb is that if you can smell it, it's probably bad for you. This can be counterintuitive for those of us who grew up associating the smell of new cars, new shoes, and a fresh coat of paint with something good. The real reason fresh paint smells is that it's releasing toxic vapors like benzene, formaldehyde, kerosene, ammonia, toluene, and xylene—known carcinogens and neurotoxins. Not all volatile organic compounds (VOCs) are alike—some are highly toxic, while others have no known health effects—but

> ### TAKE IT OFF
>
> If your painting involves stripping first, use one of the following biodegradable, water-soluble, noncaustic, nontoxic strippers. Also be sure not to strip paint with lead in it. If you're not sure, and have an old house, have it tested.
>
> CitriStrip
> Woodfinisher's Pride
> Ameristrip
> Peel Away
> RemovAll and Bio-Wash

HEALTHY NONTOXIC PAINTS

(From *The Green Guide*: WWW.THEGREENGUIDE.COM)

Brand	Natural	VOCs	Price	Contact	Use
AFM Safecoat Eggshell Zero VOC by AFM		No	$34.90/gallon	afmsafecoat.com 800-239-0321	Interior
Air-Care Coronado		No	$21/gallon	coronadopaint.com 800-883-4193	Interior
BioShield Clay Paint	Yes	No	$40/gallon	bioshieldpaint.com 800-621-2591	Interior
BioShield Solvent-Free Wall Paint	Yes	No	$34/gallon	bioshieldpaint.com 800-621-2591	Interior
Ecological Paint by Innovative Formulations Company		No	$20/gallon	innovativeformulations .com 520-628-1553	Interior/Exterior
Eco Spec by Benjamin Moore		Low	$25 to $30/ gallon	benjaminmoore.com 800-344-0400	Interior
Enviro-Safe Paint by Chem-Safe Products		No	$29.95/gallon	210-657-5321	Interior/Exterior
Genesis Odor-Free Interior Latex Flat Wall Paint by Duron		No	$26.70/gallon	duron.com 800-72-DURON	Interior
Kelly-Moore Enviro-Coat Enamel		No	$15.10/gallon	kellymoore.com 650-595-1654	Interior
Lifemaster 2000 Interior Flat Paint by ICI Dulux		No	$25/gallon	iciduluxpaints.com 216-344-8000	Interior
Safecoat Exterior Satin		Low	$35/gallon	afmsafecoat.com 800-239-0321	Exterior
Old Fashioned Milk Paint	Yes	No	$43.95/gallon	milkpaint.com 978-448-6336	Interior

most of the VOCs found in paint unfortunately fall into the former category. Most household paints today are either alkyd (solvent/oil) or water (latex/plastic/emulsion) based. Alkyd paints, which are used mostly for high-gloss jobs or to minimize mold growth in areas with high moisture, contain 32 to 42 percent VOCs, versus the 2 to 5 percent found in latex paints. However, latex paints, which are usually used for interior walls and ceilings, can contain other preservatives, fungicides, and dangerous solvents. The bottom line is that "low-VOC" paint is better than nothing, but you should buy "VOC-free," "no-VOC," or "zero-VOC" paint if you can, because they are almost completely free of carcinogenic chemicals. Try to avoid alkyd- or oil-based paints, even if they are labeled "low-VOC," in favor of latex. There are lots of "natural" paints (see page 116), which tend to cost more and are usually made from citrus and plant ingredients, milk protein, or clay. They are better for the environment because most do not use petrochemicals, produce smog, or use preservatives and biocides. But they take a lot longer to dry, are more difficult to apply, and often need to be layered in several coats. Natural paints work best in drier areas because they're less resistant to mold and mildew. Keep in mind that it takes most paints weeks to fully dry and off-gas. To be extra safe, check with the manufacturer of your paint for specifics.

work environment

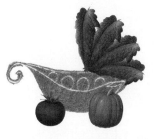

While we have friends who are lucky enough to earn their living as acrobats and musicians, this section is concerned with the more traditional work environment. There are degrees of toxicity in every job, whether you're pumping gas or faxing from your office cubicle, but they can be equally difficult in terms of figuring out how to control the flow of contaminants in your direction. Unlike in your home, it's rare to have any say about the PBDE-filled foam peeking out of the tear in your office chair. It's probably way too early to let your boss in on the big news that you're planning on procreating, but it's definitely a great time to think about getting a desk farther away from the copy machine.

One approach is to see if there is anyone who is obviously pregnant in the office who might be willing to have a conversation with a manager about some beneficial amendments to your workplace. It's unlikely he or she will replace the wall-to-wall carpeting, but you can at least keep your eyes peeled for a more inviting chair that's not being used. Choose metal over plastic when possible, and avoid vinyl at all cost.

computers

If you're like us, you sit in front of a computer almost all day long. There isn't much you can change about that if you want to keep getting a paycheck. The good news is that computers give off only small amounts of radiation that don't pose a real threat to your health. The NIOSH has done studies on workplace reproductive hazards and has found no association between video display terminals and miscarriages, low birth weights, or preterm deliveries. Other studies suggest computers might be a source of electromagnetic radiation. If you're still concerned, it has been reported that laptops with LCD screens are a little bit safer.

air

Open the windows whenever possible. Or ask your manager about what sort of ventilation system is in place. Plants can help lower certain contaminants (see the list on page 122), and who would object to some green life in fluorescent-ville? If you can't open windows, make sure to take frequent breaks. Not only will it save your back and you from other aches and pains that come from sitting in one spot all day long, but it will provide much-needed fresh air.

leaving work at work

If you or your partner are exposed to dangerous substances like toxic solvents or chemicals at work, be sure to take the following precautions to avoid bringing them home with you:

- Remove contaminated clothes, bag them, and then wash up with soap and water before putting on clean clothes to go home.
- Store street clothes in a separate area of the workplace to prevent contamination.
- Wash work clothing separately from other laundry (at work or outside of the home if possible).
- Avoid bringing contaminated clothing or other objects home. If work clothes must be brought home, transport them in a sealed bag.

For more information, contact the National Institute for Occupational Safety and Health (NIOSH): *www.cdc.gov/niosh.*

copy machines, fax machines, and printers

Most new copiers make dry copies where images are produced by electronically fusing carbon powder (toner) to paper. This powder can linger airborne for hours, acting as an irritant to those suffering from asthma or bronchitis. While some toner is carcinogenic, such a large exposure would be required that it is generally considered harmless. Rely on your nose; a strong smell could indicate the machine is malfunctioning. If you can exert any influence over the situation, ask that these big machines be kept in well-ventilated rooms. And desks should never be near copiers and printers. If yours is, ask to be moved. Plead chemical sensitivity if necessary.

supplies

No matter how bored you are at work, sniffing glue is a bad idea. Ditto Wite-Out. Most glue is filled with volatile chemicals that release toxic vapors, including some known to cause birth defects. The safest glues are white glue, yellow wood-working glue, and glue sticks. Try to find a water-based correction fluid, because it won't contain phthalates. Instead of permanent markers, use only ones that are water based. Keep in mind inhalation isn't the only issue; you can also absorb chemicals through your skin.

WASH YOUR HANDS

It almost sounds silly, but washing your hands as much as possible throughout the day, and especially before eating and drinking, can reduce your exposure to hazardous substances, not to mention regular old germs.

cleanup

You're probably not going to convince your boss to buy 100 new nontoxic desks for the office, but you might suggest to the higher-ups that they start purchasing nontoxic cleaning supplies and pest controls. They have to buy these supplies anyway.

wellness

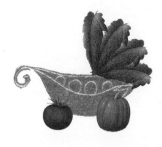

It goes without saying that right now the most important thing you can do for yourself, your fertility, and your future baby is to stop smoking, drinking alcohol, and using drugs. Pre-pregnancy is also the time to take care of anything that will be unsafe to take care of when pregnant. A good place to start is a complete checkup. Have your partner get one, too. Make sure to ask your doctor about the medications you're currently taking and their safety with regard to pregnancy. If you have any medical problems like high blood pressure or diabetes, make sure they are optimally managed by you and your doctor before getting pregnant. If you're due for a mammogram or colonoscopy, schedule them now, and avoid having X-rays once pregnant. Have all dental work (including X-rays) done before you start trying to conceive. Your dentist might tell you it's safe to have work done after the first trimester, but we feel it's better to avoid anesthesia, antibiotics, X-rays, and the possibility of infection if you can. Tooth infections can potentially complicate a pregnancy, and gum disease has been linked to premature birth, so ask your dentist how your gums are looking. Also talk to your dentist about your wisdom teeth and decide whether something should be done about them or if they can remain untouched throughout pregnancy and breastfeeding. If you really want to go the distance, you might want to consider having any silver (amalgam) fillings removed or replaced to avoid exposure to mercury

toxicity in the amalgam. Most dentists will tell you they know
remove your amalgam, but be sure to find a biological dentist
run non-mercury practices) to do the job so that you can avoid
tential exposure to mercury during the procedure.

prenatal vitamins

It's never too early to start taking a prenatal vitamin when attempting to conceive.
If one makes you feel nauseated, keep trying others, as there is a large variety on
the market. But be absolutely sure to take one that includes the maximum daily
recommended dose of folic acid (important for helping prevent neural tube defects and spina bifida). Organic prenatal vitamins do exist. The main differences
between these and more conventional vitamins is that they're vegetarian and include no filler, artificial color, or flavor.

Your care provider can advise you on certain brands, including organic ones,
but Dr. Siobhan M. Dolan, assistant professor of OB-GYN and Women's Health
at Albert Einstein College of Medicine/Montefiore Medical Center (and Deirdre's sister), recommends finding a vitamin that contains the following:

- 4,000–5,000 IU (international units) of vitamin A
- 800–1,000 mcg (1 mg) of folic acid
- 400 IU of vitamin D
- 200–300 mg of calcium
- 70 mg of vitamin C
- 1.5 mg of thiamine
- 1.6 mg of riboflavin
- 2.6 mg of pyridoxine
- 17 mg of niacinamide
- 2.2 mcg of vitamin B_{12}
- 10 mg of vitamin E
- 15 mg of zinc
- 30 mg of iron

find a care provider

If you don't already have an obstetrician or midwife in mind to deliver your baby, this is the time to start searching. This may be daunting if you haven't even given thought to what kind of birth you want to have—in a hospital with a doctor, in a birthing center with a midwife, or at home. You may not yet be totally familiar with the language of doulas, epidurals, and episiotomies. (For more, see Chapter Twelve, "Special Section—Giving Birth.")

It's hard to commit at this stage in the game. But you should because it's difficult to change courses once you're under someone's care. If you know you want to have a natural birth and you're not considered high-risk, you're best bet is probably a midwife.

Here are some thoughts we had when searching for our own practitioners. Vibe is important. Do you like the person? Does she or he make you feel comfortable? Do you know his or her birth philosophy? Hospital births are likely to include medicine and fetal monitoring. Is the birthing center your midwife works at freestanding? Or located within a hospital?

DETOX AND CLEANSING

For some women, enemas and/or colon cleanses are a part of their wellness routine. But when trying to get pregnant, this must come to a stop. Both psyllium and stool softeners are said to be okay to keep bowel movements regular (though organic prunes work just as well), but detoxification in general is not recommended while you try to get pregnant, during pregnancy, or while breastfeeding.

depression and antidepressants

If you take antidepressants and can't decide whether or not you should stop taking them when you get pregnant, you should talk to everyone on your health care team (medical doctor, therapist, midwife, psychopharmacologist) before making a decision. Depression peaks between ages twenty-five and forty-four (almost exactly overlapping with your reproductive years), and although many women (10–20%) suffer major depression during pregnancy, there is still relatively little conclusive evidence about the negative effects of antidepressants on the fetus. It's almost impossible to do a double-blind study (where neither the subjects nor the researchers know who is receiving the drug or the placebo) on pregnant women, but no studies have shown antidepressants to increase the risk of major malformations. One study showed fluoxetine (Prozac) was associated with a greater risk for minor malformations. There is conflicting evidence regarding the association between antidepressants and perinatal complications such as preterm delivery. Several, but not all, studies did show an increased risk of premature birth among pregnant women taking fluoxetine (Prozac). Withdrawal symptoms (neonatal toxicity), including jerky movements, respiratory distress, and feeding difficulties, have been reported in some babies born to mothers taking antidepressants. Studies evaluating long-term neurodevelopmental outcomes in children exposed to antidepressants in utero have shown that there is no deficit in language, behavior, or IQ. In general, there is less concern about taking medication during the second and third trimester because fetal organ development happens during the first. Make sure your care provider has the most up-to-date research there is.

We can't emphasize enough that before you stop your medication you should have a plan in place that was derived in consultation with a professional. Seeing a therapist and/or joining a support group are two good ways to begin to try to deal with symptoms. Even if you find out you're already pregnant, the most important thing is to not abruptly stop taking medication. Light therapy has also been found to be helpful for some women. "You have to weigh the decision," says Dr. Dolan. "Although I think medication would probably be the last option, there are risks to being depressed and pregnant. Some of the risk factors that can accompany depression, like inadequate weight gain, or use of drugs or alcohol, most certainly have direct negative consequences for the fetus."

Prozac Pregnancy

BY ANONYMOUS

I remember worrying about the antidepressant issue years before we even got pregnant. Prozac had literally saved my life when I started taking it, and over the ten years since then, I had tried to wean myself from it several times. But each time, I again became depressed and had to resume taking it. The only thing in life I was really afraid of was becoming depressed again. I felt that as long as I was not depressed, I could handle pretty much anything.

When my husband and I started talking about getting pregnant, I began to do some research on the safety of antidepressants during pregnancy and got very mixed results. In the end I spoke with a psychiatrist who basically said that there was some risk involved with taking antidepressants while pregnant, and also while breastfeeding. However, he also said that, given my history, the likelihood that I would again become depressed was high, and that I would be particularly susceptible to a potentially severe postpartum depression. He said that having a depressed mother could also be harmful to the development of the fetus and development of the child. He advocated stopping the medication while pregnant and then resuming it immediately postpartum, and bottle-feeding rather than breastfeeding. I appreciated his straightforward approach, but I also felt strongly about breastfeeding. I decided that I would play it by ear and try to breastfeed if I could.

When I found out that I was five weeks pregnant with my first child, I stopped the Prozac immediately. I did not feel depressed and do not remember any negative consequences at that time. Perhaps the fact that I was so ecstatic to be pregnant helped me. Then at three months pregnant we moved. This was a stressful and difficult time. I did not resume the Prozac during that pregnancy and I did not become depressed, but there were times when I felt I was skating on very thin ice and I felt scared.

One of the most insidious things about depression is the way it seems to fight against any glimmer of hope and positive thinking. When I am depressed, I think that darkness and hopelessness are the truth of life, and that anyone walking around with a smile on their face is deluded in some way. I resist the idea of taking medication and regard suicide as a much more viable solution to my pain. It doesn't matter that this makes no sense; when I am depressed, that is my reality. I remember when I first started taking medication and my depression lifted for the first time in years saying incredulously to a friend, "Is this how most people feel?" I couldn't believe how good it could feel to be alive.

Anyway, the point is that when I'm not depressed, it makes all the sense in the world to take medication—the problem is that when I am depressed, my thinking changes. Not only does it become practically impossible for me to make even a simple decision, but I start thinking medication is a bad idea. So, knowing this about myself, I was afraid. Afraid that if I became depressed and needed to get back on the meds, I might resist the idea and thus cause harm to my baby. I ended up asking several people close to me who understood depression to keep an eye on me, and if I started sounding depressed to let me know.

The birth of my first child was difficult. He was a colicky baby, and we struggled with breastfeeding. Those first few weeks were so very hard. I was crying a lot of the time, but the circumstances were so overwhelming that I could not be sure of the cause. The circumstances did gradually improve and I started to feel somewhat better, but I didn't feel good. During that time I would wonder in circles, "Am I depressed or is this just a tough time?" In some ways the circular thinking was my biggest clue that I was depressed. I was not as deeply depressed as I had been at times, and I was not thinking about suicide, but I did have thoughts that I was not a good mother, and that my son would be better off without me. I was enduring my life as I had endured so many years of it before.

With the help of friends and the recognition of my symptoms, I gradually accepted that I was depressed again. I also suspected that if anything was helping me avoid full-blown depression, it was the calming hormones released while nursing. I began to do more research and found the book *Medications and Mothers' Milk* by Dr. Thomas Hale (and his Web site, see page 222) to be very helpful. I read that once a baby reaches four months, the risks associated with nursing lessen. I was reading this at around two months and decided to wait as long as I could and then begin the medication at a lower dose than usual. I still really struggled with when to start the medication, but in my most honest moments I was aware that my mood was likely having an adverse affect on my son.

After a lot of agonizing I finally resumed the Prozac when my son was approximately five months old. I resumed the Prozac at a lower dose of 10 mg. In the past I had always taken 20 mg. I didn't notice any changes in my son, but I did begin to feel better. The better I felt, the more abundantly clear it became to me that having a happy, present mother was vitally important to my son. I don't know if it would have been better for him and me to start the meds sooner. I guess I'll never know, but I did the best I could under the circumstances.

When I became pregnant with my second child, I felt calmer about the whole process. I didn't realize I was pregnant until seven weeks and again stopped the medication as soon as I found out. My pregnancy with my daughter was a joyful time: I did not have the stress of moving that I had in my first pregnancy, and I remember feeling really great throughout. Her birth was quick and easy, I had no problem with nursing the second time, and she was a quiet, easy baby. Yet after several weeks, when I started to have dark, negative thoughts and had difficulty making decisions, I knew I was skating on thin ice again. When my daughter was four months old, I resumed the Prozac once again at 10 mg. I struggled a bit with the decision, but nothing like the first time.

I do not know what the right choice is for other women. It would be a lot easier if there were a clear-cut right and wrong. I love that I breastfed my children, and I think that nursing actually helped provide a buffer to depression. And, for whatever reason (hormones probably), I seemed to be okay while I was pregnant. The hardest part of the whole process for me was deciding whether and when to restart the medications. I hope this can be of some help to other mothers who are wrestling with this issue. It is not an easy one, but one thing that is clear to me is that I make the best decisions and I am the best mother to my children when I am not depressed.

pre-pregnancy testing

About 150,000 babies are born each year with birth defects. Several thousand different birth defects have been identified, but the causes of about 60 to 70 percent of them are still unknown. Schedule a pre-pregnancy visit with your health care provider to decide what pre-pregnancy tests are appropriate for you. A pre-pregnancy visit is especially crucial for women with medical problems like diabetes, high blood pressure, and epilepsy, all of which can affect pregnancy. Women with poorly controlled diabetes are several times more likely than women without diabetes to have a baby with a serious birth defect. However, if your blood sugar levels are well controlled before pregnancy, you are almost as likely to have a healthy baby as a woman without diabetes.

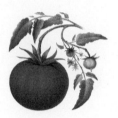

GENETIC TESTING

For in-depth definitions of genetic disorders go to *www.geneticalliance.org*. A pre-pregnancy visit will generally include testing for the following:

1. Sickle-cell anemia (African Americans)
2. Thalassemia (Mediterraneans and Southeast Asians)
3. Cystic fibrosis (Northern Europeans, Ashkenazi Jews; optional for African Americans and Asians)
4. Fragile X syndrome
5. Ashkenazi Jewish genetic diseases (a group of rare disorders that occur more frequently in people of Eastern European Jewish heritage than in the general population)

My Virtuous Life

BY LEXY ZISSU

This is a pep talk. Once upon a time before I got pregnant I lived happily with three close friends: Advil, wine, and coffee. Every morning when I woke up, I made two shots of espresso, heated organic skim milk in stainless steel on the stove, stirred in some brown sugar, and sat down with my boyfriend for as long as time would permit, sipping away, coming alive, waking up. Life without coffee wasn't imaginable. I'd begun every day like that since I was fourteen and stayed out all night when visiting a friend in Paris (how glam) and met the sunrise with my first grand crème. The ritual changed from time to time—in high school I drank it light and extremely sweet out of blue-and-white paper cups from a deli on the corner; in college I guzzled weak, flavored imitations of real coffee out of a plastic thermos that didn't smell so great but if you downed all sixteen ounces sort of did the trick. When I first started working, I added an extra dose of caffeine—a cup of Earl Grey tea—in the afternoons. But the true fact of my relationship with coffee never wavered: I had to start my day with it or else I was totally useless.

It's less socially acceptable to say the same goes for wine and Advil, but essentially this was also true for me. Wine (could there be anything more organic? It's heaven brought about by grapes) was there for me at the end of pretty much every day. Not a huge amount. But enough to savor, roll around my mouth, take the edge off. Crisp whites and Prosecco bubbles in the summer. Heavy, earthy reds to match the fall and winter. A glass of wine was easily my favorite guest at early Sunday dinners. It was something I truly looked forward to daily. And what was I doing with all of that Advil? Well, until I was twenty-six years old, I pretty much didn't lift a finger or exercise. Around then I started doing a huge amount of yoga. I love it. I now live for it with a coffee/wine/Advil sort of fervor, but it makes me sore. Very sore. Heating pads are great, so are hot baths if you have the time and a clean-ish bathtub, but Advil is really an amazing thing. So I succumbed. A little too often.

When I started trying to get pregnant, I gave up all three cold turkey. NB: this is not the smartest way to go about giving things up. I should have weaned. Withdrawal headaches abounded, mainly from the caffeine. Not being able to drink put a huge crimp in my social life, sad but true. I missed the easy camaraderie of meeting friends for drinks, a glass of wine. Seltzer with lime just isn't as fun. And my shoulders ached. After two weeks of this, I discovered I wasn't pregnant and went immediately back on coffee, then wine. The first cup was insane. I was high as a kite. It made me realize how sad it was that I usually barely felt something so strong. The wine, however, was a pure delight. As it always is. Deirdre told me I was crazy, that if I came off, I should just stay off.

The next time off was a bit easier. I toyed with decaf teas and coffees, which do have a bit of caffeine in them. But before I had a chance to experiment with further weaning, I was off for good. I was pregnant. Staying off all three when actually pregnant is comparatively easy. I wish I had known that. Your body takes over. You don't really want any of it. Okay, so an Advil would be just lovely when your lower back is about to fall off your body because it aches so much, but no matter. I did just fine without.

fitness

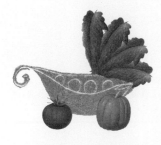

Everyone knows pregnancy is no longer an excuse to sit around and eat ice cream. Women have realized that an active nine months generally translates into a more comfortable pregnancy and faster postpartum recovery. It's not uncommon to see women well into their third trimester with yoga mats tucked under their arms, or bumps on the next StairMaster over. If you're not exactly a gym fan, now is a good time to start thinking about finding a low-impact form of exercise you can tolerate, so that your body has time to get used to it. Picking up something new when you're already pregnant is potentially dangerous, not to mention less likely to stick, especially when you're suffering from nausea and the other lovely perks of your first trimester. And when you're pregnant, exhaustion does feel like a legitimate excuse not to work out. Pre-pregnancy is a great time to get in shape. That said, now is also not a good time to overdo it. Really serious workout-aholics may have body fat levels that are low enough to negatively affect fertility. This isn't a time to be marathon training; this is about general heart-healthy activity.

If you play a sport that involves bumping and falling (soccer, hockey, softball), this may be your last chance for a while. These activities are too risky for pregnant women. Though many longtime runners jog all the way through pregnancy without issue, New York–based pregnancy fitness expert Janette Wallis says better options include walking, stationary bike riding, weight lifting, and yoga. Pre-pregnancy is a great time to work on your stomach muscles, especially the lower abs. Abdominal work is harder to do when pregnant. "You want to have a strong pelvic floor that gives support to the uterus before you get pregnant," says Wallis. Ideally, you want to enter a pregnancy strong all over. This will help you carry the extra weight.

If you've worked out seriously over the years and want to continue, but aren't getting the go-ahead you'd like from, say, your in-laws or midwife or obstetrician, we recommend a book called *Exercising Through Your Pregnancy* by Dr. James F. Clapp III. Dr. Clapp has done extensive research on vigorous workouts during pregnancy. His findings made Lexy feel comfortable enough to continue standing on her head during yoga for many months (though she did lay off kicking up into handstands and jumping back into chattarunga), and Deirdre feel comfortable enough to pick up her forty-pound bull terrier, Harriet, at will.

One thing to keep in mind, specifically if you're exercising outdoors in a big city, is to try choosing a spot with a high concentration of trees; the air will be cleaner.

swimming

What could be better than floating weightless when pregnant? Swimming is a low-impact, wonderful form of exercise. We wish we could tell every pre-pregnant woman to take it up immediately, and to lap her way through her nine months without reservation. But we can't. Skin is the body's largest organ, and if it can absorb the medicine in a nicotine or birth control patch, it can absorb chlorine. Chlorine is a persistent organic pollutant, and a seriously toxic chemical. Even the fumes are bad news. A study published in the June 2003 issue of *Occupational and Environmental Medicine* demonstrated that the layer of chlorine gases hovering just above the water in a pool have the potential to damage the lungs and cause asthma if the levels are high enough. Chlorine that stings the eyes can also "sting" the sensitive tissue of the lungs. Chlorine—even in tap water—has been linked (in studies in the United States, Canada, and Norway) to higher risks of miscarriage, stillbirths, and increased incidences of bladder and colon cancer. Higher levels of cancers are found in swimmers. We are exposed to much higher dosages of chlorine during a swim than in drinking or showering in chlorinated water.

If you choose to swim now and throughout your pregnancy, try to find a less-chlorinated (or otherwise disinfected) private pool, an outdoor pool, a lake, or maybe even a saltwater pool. If your only option is an indoor pool, look for one in a space with windows that can be opened for ventilation. If not, try to find one in a building with very high ceilings. And avoid swimming daily.

your partner

Working out is not just about you. You want your future baby's daddy to be in good shape as well, but not to the detriment of his fertility. If bike riding's his thing, he should know that there have been a number of studies questioning its long-term effects on sperm production. Average amounts of biking are not a problem, but those who bike hundreds of miles a week should be aware that a combination of tight biking shorts and prolonged contact with a hard bike seat can considerably diminish the capacity to produce sperm. Stopping or cutting back on cycling will help reverse negative effects. So can pointing the saddle slightly downward, using a wider saddle, wearing padded bike shorts, and taking frequent rests during long rides.

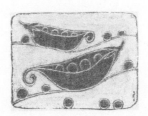

play

When trying to conceive, it may feel like all your downtime is spent charting your temperature, surfing fertility Web sites, and standing on your head. You may not have as much time to devote to your old hobbies, but here are some thoughts on your new one.

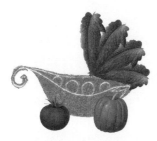

fertility and food

When looking for some help with fertility from your general diet, many advocate sticking to fiber-rich, low-fat vegetables and grains and taking a pass on fatty, cholesterol-laden meat and dairy products. There are plenty of nonscientific theories about the powers of fertility in foods like shark's fin and figs, and some people think spicy food increases sexual potency by raising blood pressure, but there's no proof. However, there is some scientific proof that eating foods rich in certain vitamins can help. Yams are thought to be good for female reproductive organs, and oysters are thought to help because they are packed with zinc, which plays a role in semen and testosterone production

> ### SLUGGISH SPERM?
>
> According to Susan Allport, author of *The Queen of Fats: Why Omega-3's Were Removed from the Western Diet and What We Can Do to Replace Them,* there are some natural alternatives for boosting your fertility. If your partner's sperm are less than sprightly, it can help him to start taking omega-3 fatty acids (up to 12 grams a day).

and in ovulation and fertility. But don't go crazy—you don't want to go over the recommended dietary allowance of zinc a day (9 mg), because too much can actually reduce your fertility and make you nauseated (which never helps in the sex department).

Net Loss

BY DEIRDRE DOLAN

I had a dream I was bleeding. Not from a cut or a wound, but from a fertilized embryo digging into my uterine wall. I was dreaming about implantation spotting, and I knew why. For a few precious minutes, even though I was fast asleep, I was letting myself feel what it would be like to be pregnant. It was a feeling I'd been looking forward to for a year, and it felt pretty great. The dream was a reprieve from my waking life, where all time was divided into the two weeks after I ovulated, and the two after I got my period. People have waited longer for things, to get their braces off, or for a new season of *The Sopranos*, but ten months was starting to feel like forever.

Actively waiting for something is a huge bummer. Every month I was newly surprised the waiting was going to continue. We were so sure it would happen right away that the realization at about month five that it wasn't only seemed like a sign of more bad news to come. I tried action mode—was there anything else I could do (on top of giving up caffeine, alcohol, sugar, and dairy) to make it happen? I tried bugging my gynecologist for an explanation. But the fact is, if you've been trying for only five months, all a busy Manhattan doctor's going to tell you is good luck.

My friend Anna told me about a Chinese herbalist and acupuncturist she'd seen for fertility. Anna is positive she helped her get pregnant by getting rid of her chronic stomachache through acupuncture, diet, and herbs (see page 70). I called the doctor and made an appointment. I didn't have anything as tangible wrong with me, but it was a relief to be doing something.

At our weekly appointment, the doctor gave me acupuncture, checked my pulse, examined my tongue, and reviewed a food diary of everything I'd eaten that week.

She reviewed my basal body temperature (BBT) chart and wrote me a prescription for fertility herbs from Chinatown.

I was a model patient for a few months. I wrote down every Snickers I snuck and felt pretty can-do buying, boiling, and drinking bag after bag of foul-tasting herbs. I also obsessed about my BBT, a daily ritual that made me feel like I had some control. I took my temperature every morning like I was being graded. If the number was too high or low, I felt bad; within the appropriate range, I felt good. I knew it was ridiculous to get emotionally invested in my body temperature, but I couldn't help it. I couldn't even tell if I was really feeling bad when I thought I was because it still felt too early to justify feeling bad.

Rule number one with pregnancy is avoid stress, and one day it dawned on me that what I'd hoped would be a soothing organic antidote to my hurried OB-GYN was stressing me out more than doing nothing. I stopped going to the acupuncturist, and suddenly I was back to square one.

Then I made a big mistake. I turned to the Internet.

I tiptoed in, mostly aware it was a minefield waiting. It was always during the second two weeks of my cycle that I'd get impatient and start typing random words into Google like "cervix" and "position" and "newly pregnant" so I could find out if, say, mine was in pregnant position. Then I'd scroll through the more intriguing of the 23,400 links that appeared before me, learn everything there was to know about something called an incompetent cervix, and just like that, another hour of my life would be gone forever.

On most subjects, but especially the mystery of pregnancy, the Internet can provide absolutely any information you need to find. Itchy palms? Puffy eyes? More thirsty than usual? It didn't take much for me to start a search. I had no idea what pregnancy would feel like, so if I noticed anything irregular, I tried to turn it into the confirmation I wanted. All I had to do was find one pregnant person in cyberspace who also happened to feel a little thirsty on day 26 of her cycle, and I could relax into a state of false hopefulness for the rest of the day.

There are three main types of pregnancy sites—infertility, fertility, and medical. The infertility sites (with letdown names like Vintage Uterus, My Eggs Are Cooked, Panic Womb, Knocked Down, Wasted Birth Control, and Barren Mare) are where women blog their own experience of not getting pregnant. They have an unapologetically pissed-off tone and made me feel despairing, hopeless, and sucked into other people's misery. Some women sounded like spoiled ten-year-olds, and some sounded bitter for very good reason. I found it too hard to figure out where I fit in on the spectrum.

The fertility sites, with their sunny outlooks and sometimes overwhelming religious fervor, were even worse. These sites are full of posts from eternally hopeful women who are constantly sprinkling "baby dust" on everyone, abbreviating words, talking about their "dear husbands," and "baby dancing" instead of having sex. Spending a Sunday night in a chat room with a bunch of English women posting words of support: "Well done you, Jacksmommy!" or advice: "Don't forget the cold showers to wake up the wrigglers!" or neither: "Oh blimey, I feel sick, I knew I shouldn't have eaten the corned beef!" is kind of culturally interesting. But it's more like group-therapy reality TV.

I had enough sense to avoid the medical Web sites completely. Had I not, I'm sure I would have diagnosed myself as having everything from hostile cervical mucus to premature ovarian failure (even if it doesn't affect women under forty).

I knew it was time to step away from the computer, so I made an appointment with a fertility specialist. I felt a huge relief after the first appointment. The ball was no longer in my court. I could stop freaking out about not being able to figure out what was wrong with me. He gave me an exam and said nothing seemed wrong, but that if I wanted to up my chances, I could take Clomid to stimulate ovulation. If I took a low dose, it would only increase my chance of multiple births by 6 percent. I started taking it, and now I'm pregnant. Maybe it happened at last because I finally stopped worrying about it, or because science came to the rescue. But either way, I've finally got something new to wait for, and this time, I know exactly how long it'll take.

fertility and herbs

We've talked to lots of women who found acupuncture and Chinese herbs to be a big help when trying to get pregnant. Acupuncture is thought to help to regulate your system and get things that might not be working back in shape by normalizing the production of hormones. Herbs are also considered by some to be good for getting your blood flowing to your reproductive organs, which can help improve the health and function of your ovaries and uterus. There is some debate about how well this works, but as long as you see a trained acupuncturist, there is also no harm giving it a shot. Studies have shown that acupuncture with in vitro fertilization raises the chance of pregnancy from 20 to 40 percent.

ACUPUNCTURE TESTIMONIAL
by Deirdre's friend Anna

Right when my husband and I started trying to get pregnant, my body seemed to shut down. I started having terrible stomachaches accompanied by bloating and constipation. The cycles of my period, which were normally 28 to 32 days, slowed down to 60 or even 80 days. It was taking me 40 days to ovulate. I went to my gynecologist and she suggested going back on the pill to regulate my cycles or to try Clomid. Neither option seemed to address what to me seemed like a systemic problem—not just a fertility issue. So I went to see a Chinese doctor recommended by a friend. She gave me a complete evaluation (through an extensive conversation about medical history and general habits) and gave me a diagnosis best summarized as "stuck." The symptoms had all started after a period of extreme stress, and since I tend to handle stress by going into a kind of deep freeze, she explained that my body had shut down. To get things moving again she put me on a new diet, which included much more protein (I hadn't eaten much red meat before), much less sugar and alcohol, and less water (I was drinking too much before, which can hamper digestion). I also started on a regimen of awful-tasting herbs and acupuncture. Within a month my stomach symptoms were much better; within three months the cycle of my periods was speeding up, so that every cycle was 15 days shorter than the last one. Six months in, my stomach was fine, my cycle was back to normal, and I got pregnant.

herbs to avoid while pregnant or trying to get pregnant

Some herbs are contraindicated when pregnant because they are thought to have an influence on the uterus. These include: barberry, bloodroot, calamus, cascara sagrada, fennel, goldenseal, juniper, lavender, licorice root, male fern, mayapple, mistletoe, passionflower, pennyroyal, periwinkle, poke root, rhubarb, St. John's wort, tansy, wild cherry, wormwood, and yarrow.

travel vaccinations

It's generally recommended that you wait at least four weeks between having a vaccination and getting pregnant, but make sure to run this by your doctor. After live vaccines, some experts recommend waiting around three months. So if you are planning a holiday to a high-risk area, use contraception for at least a month after having vaccinations.

The Old-Fashioned Way

BY STACEY KOFF

My partner, Margie, and I walk hand in hand into our doctor's Santa Monica office. With her free hand, Margie pushes our daughter, Anabelle, in her stroller. In my free hand, I hold an oversized canister containing the sperm of an anonymous donor. It isn't sexy or hot—more awkward and humiliating—but loving in its own way.

The waiting room is full of women reading magazines while they wait for their Pap smears, pelvic exams, or news that they are safe to go home to begin trying to conceive. I approach the front desk and let the receptionist know that I'm here for an insemination. She asks me to sign in and I do before turning to find a seat next to Margie and Anabelle. I am three feet away from the desk when the receptionist calls out, "Do you have the sperm?" The room gets suddenly smaller and more intimate. Immediately, yet inconspicuously, *Cosmopolitan, Vogue,* and *FitPregnancy* magazines lower just enough for gazes to fall on me. "Yes," I say with an obvious look of embarrassment—what the hell did she think was in the enormous canister under my arm?

In the cold small white examination room Margie stands above me holding my hand as our doctor pokes and prods at my cervix to try to help us do what so many others can do in the privacy of their bedroom, bathroom, kitchen table, or restroom stall in a sleazy bar. We, too, can conceive; the means are distinct, but the end is the same. Anabelle is sitting in her stroller eating Pirate's Booty and kicking her legs up and down. She watches the doctor work diligently to help us give her a baby brother or sister. Every once in a while she tosses a piece of Booty at my legs in the stirrups, laughs, and looks up at us. She is heaven sent. Somehow, in this freezing, sterile room, I feel at home, so perfect and hopeful knowing that there is no other way that I would like this to happen. That all the love in the world is in this room with me, and that our hope and love will help us conceive.

After some twinges of abdominal pain and a good shot of semen into my uterus, we leave the doctor's office and get in the car. I have my seat as far back as it can be reclined, to try to keep every drop of sperm inside me. I am lying back and talking to Anabelle in her car seat, when Margie takes a sharp turn toward home and we hear a crash from the trunk of our car. This is followed by a loud hissing noise, as dry ice starts to fill the car like a bad horror movie. We pull into a gas station, laughing, and open the trunk to assess the damage. The canister is empty, but I reseal the lid so that we can return it to the bank from whence it came. The fourth insemination is over. I eat healthily, take my prenatals, wait, and continue loving on my girls.

We know that this is our fate for a while. We know that even though we make love the night before and after insemination, it will not get us pregnant. We know that someday after many inseminations and embarrassing mishaps with sperm and waiting rooms, we will conceive and give Anabelle a sibling. Two weeks later, I get my period and we begin thinking and preparing for the process yet again.

STACEY KOFF is a school administrator in Los Angeles.

beauty

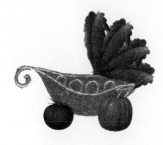

Beauty products smell good, make us look pretty, and promise instant perfection—flawless skin, thick, shiny hair, solid nails. Unfortunately most are loaded with chemicals linked to birth defects, carcinogens, ingredients derived from nonrenewable petroleum, and preservatives that can end up in breast tissue. The Environmental Working Group says 89 percent of the ingredients in everyday products aren't tested for safety. Which is why—especially when pregnant—organic beauty products are the way to go. But there's a catch: our government doesn't regulate personal products the way it regulates food (though there have been some advances made recently, and hopefully more to come). This means that any shampoo company can slap the label "organic" or "natural" on its product. In the absence of government regulation, the genuine organic- and biodynamic-beauty-product producers (a significant minority) have tried to find a way to differentiate themselves. Many of them are European companies and adhere to comparatively strict European standards. Several trustworthy merchants have also stepped up to help consumers locate the purest products possible, including Kirstin Binder, who runs the very cool organic beauty Web site, *SaffronRouge.com*. Binder has a degree in phytotherapy (the study of herbal medicine). The products on her site have passed rigorous qualifying standards, guaranteeing that no synthetic chemicals, fertilizers, pesticides, sewage sludge, or genetically modified organisms were used to make them, and that both animal welfare and the environment were respected. Compared with the large number of so-called organic beauty products available on the market today, it's noteworthy that Binder found only a handful of product lines that met her standards. These include Primavera, Weleda, Dr. Hauschka, John Masters Organics, Jurlique, Pangea Organics, Lavera, and Sympathical Formulas. Binder's site ships anywhere, bringing organic beauty to people who might have trouble finding it locally.

product purge

When thinking about getting pregnant, or trying to get pregnant, we urge you to spend a few hours in your bathroom. Sift through your products. Read the labels. Compare and contrast the ingredients in your bottles with our what-to-avoid list on page 77.

It's not easy to discard all of your hard-learned and reliable beauty secrets overnight. If there is something you absolutely can't live without, don't sweat it. Lexy honestly believes that if Kiehl's Crème with Silk Groom had existed when she was in high school (to tame the frizzy monster on top of her head), her social life might have been significantly better. And so now as an adult she clings to its magical properties even though it includes parabens (see page 78). Her rationalization? It's on her (dead) hair, not her (living) skin. She's much more willing to give up products that linger on her skin for hours at a time (good-bye beloved Clearasil). For Deirdre, it would be next to impossible to abandon the Lancôme face powder that keeps her pale Irish skin a secret, but it's the only makeup she uses on a daily basis.

When we first started reading about beauty products, we wanted to toss everything in our bathrooms. But this doesn't make good environmental sense. If there are things you now deem overly chemical because you're trying to get pregnant, give them to friends who aren't. Or use them up and replace with more natural versions. Keep in mind, however, that when using new organic products, especially those with high concentrations of essential oils, you may break out. Just because plants are natural doesn't mean they won't irritate you, and switching to new products often provokes rashes. Stick it out. In time your body will adjust.

Consider everything you use from soaps to shampoos to face masks. Unless it's a can't-survive-without item, think twice about the things you leave on the longest—eye cream, sunblock, and nail polish. If you wear a lot of lipstick, make the switch to an organic or purer version. Women eat six to twelve pounds of lipstick in their lifetime. If you're married to your favorite color, at least wipe it off before eating or drinking. If you can see it on your water glass, you're swallowing it.

open wide

Don't forget toothpaste. There are two choices here, both up to you. The first is fluoride or no fluoride. It helps reduce tooth decay, but it's a toxin. Many people think they get plenty of fluoride in their tap water; they don't need extra in their toothpaste. The American Dental Association says that the concentration found in "optimally fluoridated water" is nontoxic. In 2005, eleven unions representing more than 7,000 Environmental Protection Agency workers called for a moratorium on programs to add fluoride to drinking water, citing a possible cancer risk. This all came about among allegations that a Harvard University dentistry professor had downplayed research showing an increased risk of bone cancer for boys who drink fluoridated tap water. The second choice is buying a conventional versus a natural brand. Even if you're going the fluoride route, there are reasons to buy a natural toothpaste. Conventional brands pump their pastes with chemicals to try to deliver on their promises of white smiles and tartar control. Many of these cleansers, sweeteners (including saccharin and aspartame), foaming agents, and preservatives are on our to-avoid list (see page 77). Maybe you're not swallowing when you brush (as a small child might), but some of these unsavory, possibly carcinogenic ingredients are getting into your system, especially as they slosh around your tender (maybe bleeding) gums. Most natural toothpaste brands (like Tom's of Maine) come in fluoridated and unfluoridated versions. The purest, like Weleda and Vita-Myr, only come without.

DON'T CHEW ON THIS

Slick dental flosses are often coated with a type of Teflon called PTFE (polytetrafluoroethylene). Plain, unwaxed varieties are your best bets.

pass the soap

Pretty soon hand washing is going to become more important than ever. You don't want to get sick when pregnant, and you won't want any of your newborn's visitors getting her sick either. Hospital workers and germophobes everywhere swear by Purell and other antibacterials, but recent studies suggest plenty of hand washing with plain old soap and water works just as well. And it turns out it's better for you, too. In fact, U.S. health experts and scientists have asked the FDA to pass restrictions on antibacterial soaps, citing evidence that shows soap handles bacteria as well as antimicrobial chemical additives. Their concern is that the overuse of the antibacterial bubbles and gels will create stronger, antibacterial-resistant bacteria.

skin R$_x$

If you have been using any prescription skin medication, you'll most likely want to stop using it now. Your dermatologist should advise. Lexy gave up a topical steroid she had been using for excema, and Deirdre gave up a similar steroid for her psoriasis. Drugs like Accutane are considered extremely unsafe during pregnancy. Just remember that some doctors have no problem recommending products we consider dangerous. If this is confusing, it was for us, too. Second opinions as well as the Web sites on page 77 helped us to make up our minds about the safest possible alternative solutions.

Ask your partner to make a similar edit of his products; things like Rogaine and hair dye aren't so great for his sperm, either.

SAFE PRODUCTS BOOKMARKED

- The Environmental Working Group, *www.ewg.org,* offers a searchable database, Skin Deep, with an impressive range of beauty products. It rates cosmetics in terms of how safe they are, specifically taking pregnancy into account.
- The German Web site *www.kontrollierte-naturkosmetik.de* lists the cosmetic companies (in English) that adhere to strict BDIH (Association of German Industries and Trading Firms) organic and biodynamic guidelines for certified natural cosmetics. These are extremely helpful when you're combing through the products you currently use. It is disheartening to learn how far ahead of us Europe is in terms of regulating cosmetics.
- Campaign for Safe Cosmetics: *www.safecosmetics.org*
- Children's Health Environmental Coalition: *www.checnet.org*

THE TOP FOURTEEN COSMETIC INGREDIENTS TO AVOID
(WITH SPECIAL THANKS TO SUSAN WEST KURZ, PRESIDENT OF DR. HAUSCHKA)

ANTIBACTERIALS	Soap and water are just as good as the antibacterial agents that create drug-resistant bacteria that are found in these cleansers and other cosmetic products.
COAL TAR	Coal tar chemicals are found in makeup and many hair dyes. Certain colors are probable carcinogens; others have been found to cause cancer when applied to skin. Nothing you want your fetus basting in.
DIETHANOLAMINE (DEA)	This chemical, and its compounds, which include triethanolamine (TEA), is found in shampoos and other products and is suspected to be a carcinogen.
ETHOXYLATES	Many cosmetic ingredients are created with the help of these toxic petroleum-derived surfactants. Polyethylene glycols are among the most common, and each is identified on labels as "PEG," followed by a number. There are literally hundreds of PEGs on your cosmetic labels. (BDIH Certified Natural Cosmetics aren't allowed to contain ethoxylated ingredients.)

FORMALDEHYDE	Found in way too many cosmetics, from mascara to nail polish, formaldehyde is thought to be a carcinogen according to both the EPA and the National Toxicology Program. If you're carefully reading labels, formaldehyde in its liquid state is found in the ingredients quaternium-15, DMDM hydantoin, and diazolidinyl urea. These can be absorbed through both the nails and the skin.
GLYCOL ETHERS	Some glycol ethers are thought to be reproductive hazards and can be found in everything from deodorant to perfume. When trying to find out if your favorite product contains these industrial solvents, look for ingredients with methyl in them, as well as DPGME, EGME, EGPE, EGEE, DEGBE, and PGME.
METALS: LEAD AND MERCURY	These are brain and nervous system toxins, hormone disrupters, and carcinogens to be avoided when trying to get pregnant, when pregnant, and beyond. Lead can be found as lead acetate in makeup and hair dye and be absorbed into the skin. Mercury is sometimes allowed (in very small doses) as a preservative.
PARABENS (METHYL-, ETHYL-, BUTYL-, AND PROPYLPARABEN)	As a group, parabens are the most widely used cosmetic preservatives. They were banned in European cosmetics but are still allowed by the FDA. There is growing evidence that they mimic estrogen, which disrupts hormonal activity. A recent finding of high levels of parabens in breast tumors has spurred U.S. consumer protection groups to lobby the FDA against their use.
PETROLATUM	This is all over the place, found in many cosmetics, including lipsticks, creams (and baby ointments), petroleum jelly, and even eye shadow. Some people with sensitive skin say it causes allergic reactions. The reasons to avoid are twofold: it's derived from petroleum, a nonrenewable resource. And organic beauty folks say it doesn't allow skin to breathe.
PHENYLENEDIAMINE (PPD)	PPD can be found in hair dye (and is also known as peroxide, amino, or oxidation dye). It causes skin and respiratory irritations and is thought to be carcinogenic. It's widely banned in Europe.
PHTHALATE (DIETHYL, DIETHYL HEXYL, DIBUTYL PHTHALATE)	A phthalate is a toxic petroleum derivative that has been associated with disorders of sexual maturation in girls and birth defects in boys, and has been found to produce liver cancer in lab animals. Phthalates are widely used to keep plastics flexible but are also the active ingredient that helps make cosmetics, nail polish, hair sprays, gels, and lotions soft and resilient. Diethyl phthalate is also frequently used as a fixative in fragrances, particularly synthetic fragrances. When phthalates are used in a cosmetic's fragrance, they are not required to be listed on the label, so there is no way to tell if a cosmetic contains them without contacting the manufacturer. Try to find fragrance-free products or ones scented with pure essential oils. BDIH products don't allow phthalates. (For more on phthalates in your home, see page 36.)

SILICONES (SI-, TRI-, DIMETHICONE)	Though silicone in itself is not toxic and is in fact a necessary nutrient and found as silica in the environment, the process of making silicone for cosmetics often involves use of synthetic carriers like butyl glycol. It's not easy to determine the carrier material from the label, so it's best to steer clear of all silicones. BDIH products don't allow silicones with synthetic carriers.
SODIUM LAURYL SULFATE (SLS)	This substance makes everything from shampoo to bubble bath to toothpaste foam. The Cosmetic Ingredient Review (the industry experts who test the safety of ingredients) reported that it caused enough changes in mouse skin to warrant further study. The Environmental Working Group says avoid SLS whenever possible.
TOLUENE	Yet another toxic ingredient found in nail polish, toluene can irritate both the skin and the respiratory tract. It can also cause liver damage (though you'd have to use an extreme amount).

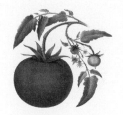

CHAPTER SIX

special section— getting a late start

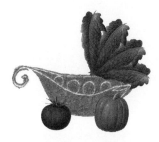

If you had a positive pregnancy test before you started transforming, the following cheat sheet can help you catch up quickly.

1. food

Adopt a whole foods diet. Give up caffeine and alcohol. Eat as much organic food as possible, training yourself to pay attention to the most and least toxic items. Meat is high on the food chain and tends to contain more toxins; vegetables are lower. Make sure you're eating a varied diet and getting plenty of protein, folic acid, calcium, and whole grains. Avoid packaged foods. Drink plenty of fluids, preferably water.

2. water

Test your water for contaminants, then purchase the appropriate antidote. Install a showerhead filter as well; this will reduce your exposure to chlorine, among other chemicals found in municipal water. (While in the bathroom, get rid of that vinyl shower curtain; it isn't a plastic you want around your growing baby. It's a known carcinogen—which contains phthalates—petroleum derivatives that have been associated with disorders of sexual maturation in girls and birth defects in boys.) Drink out of glass, not plastic.

3. air

Throw open your windows at work, in the car, and at home. Houses today are made to seal hot and cold air in, but unfortunately this also keeps many environmental pollutants in. If you're unable to access fresh air at work, get up from your desk and take periodic walks around the block. This is also good for your body and any pregnancy aches and pains you might already be experiencing.

4. kitchen

Stop using nonstick or Teflon pans, which are known to cause cancer. Cast-iron cookware is the way to go. Glass and stainless steel are equally safe to cook with. Store your food in glass instead of plastic.

5. beauty products

Do a quick run-through of the products you're using. The chemicals in them can harm you and your growing baby—no more zit cream, no more alpha hydroxies, remove nail polish. There is no government regulation of organic beauty products, so you never really know if an organic product is truly organic, but there are certain brands known to be more pure than others (see pages 74 and 77).

6. testing

Test for home contaminants. Purchase a carbon monoxide monitor. Cover cracked lead paint with fresh paint (a zero-VOC version), which is safer and cheaper than having it removed. Radon levels can easily be reduced with adequate ventilation.

7. cleaning products and insecticides

Replace all toxic cleaning products with lung- and earth-friendlier versions. Even if you're not the one cleaning, residual chemicals from these products linger in your home and are potentially very harmful to your unborn child. Apply the same approach to fertilizers, herbicides, and pesticides in your garden. If you have an insect infestation, use safer insecticides like nontoxic traps.

8. vitamins

Get on a prenatal vitamin. There are organic versions that are dye-free and contain fewer and more natural ingredients. Just make sure they have the right dosages of everything you need, especially folic acid to help prevent neural tube defects.

9. renovation

Resist the urge to renovate your home or a room for a baby nursery unless you're not living in the space you're renovating. Construction materials, paint, dust, caulk, and glues all contain dangerous toxins you don't want to be breathing when pregnant. If you must renovate, make sure to research each material being used, and work with a contractor who is willing to use nontoxic or less toxic products.

10. furniture detox

It's too expensive to buy all new furniture and mattresses, but do replace any crumbling foam or torn couch or chair cushions. The flame retardants in these foams have been found in house dust, umbilical cord blood, and breast milk.

PART TWO *growing*

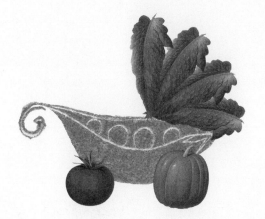

INTRODUCTION

Being newly pregnant—before you tell people, before your belly swells, maybe even before you feel sick—is completely surreal. Your secret. You go to the post office, to work, or to the movies and no one around you knows, but in your mind you're screaming, "I'm pregnant!!" It's easy to think something so small doesn't count yet. But it does. A positive pregnancy test means it's time to act like you're training for the Baby Olympics, organic style. Everyone knows having a real, live baby is a huge amount of work. But you have a job to do when you're pregnant, too. You're hosting your future child. Everything you eat, drink, breathe, and slather on should be as pure as possible to give your baby the chance to be as healthy as can be. If you didn't take the time to purge your body and your surroundings before you got pregnant, check out Part 1 and play catch-up now. Meanwhile, start thinking of yourself as a host, or a gardener, or a filter—whatever image works best for you. In this section we'll walk you through how to be the best filter possible, in all areas of your life. As always, if you can't do 100 percent of what we suggest, do what you can—something is better than nothing. And don't forget to enjoy. And take pictures. The minute you give birth you won't believe you were ever that big.

CHAPTER SEVEN

food

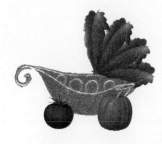

Eating becomes an adventure when you're pregnant. And it can sometimes feel like a chore. The nice thing is, it's natural to want to eat better when you have a growing guest inside you. A good diet is better for you, too. Conditions like anemia and preeclampsia are more common among pregnant women who ignore their diets. A healthy diet also helps with less serious pregnancy issues like morning sickness (a full stomach can keep nausea at bay), exhaustion, and constipation. Most doctors and midwives won't tell you to eat for two—the going thought is to add roughly 300 calories per day, and gain about twenty to thirty pounds when pregnant. It's not like you're suddenly eating that much more; it just feels like you are because each morsel is scrutinized and every bite counts. Empty calories like sugar and throwaway carbs are no longer a very good option. Without getting too obsessive, everything you eat should be contributing to your child's physical development. If you've already taken steps to transform to a more organic (preferably nonpackaged food) diet, great. If not, this is the time. Even if it's not your preferred way of eating, what's nine months if it leads to a healthier baby?

We think that a whole foods diet filled with protein, dairy, whole grains, vitamin C–rich foods, ample amounts of fruits and vegetables, and all things rich in iron is the way to go. It will require some thought on your part—grocery shopping and cooking your own food—to make sure that what crosses your lips has the highest nutrient content possible. But it's not any more effort than, say, getting up in the middle of the night to feed your baby will be. There's no choice there. And we think there really is no choice here, either. So without breaking things down into the number of ounces of cheese you'll require daily, we just want to encourage you to eat well. Use common sense, and try to cover all the food groups in a given day. Double up where you can to make it easier—pork loin is both a nice, lean protein and contains a lot of iron. Listen to your body. There will be days when you don't get all the leafy greens you could use, but don't fret about it. As *This Organic Life* author Joan Dye Gussow once told us, "I don't eat two from column A and one from B. I basically believe that if you eat a diet of whole foods and you don't add too much fat, salt, and sugar to it, you can't not be well nourished."

As soon as you start thinking about everything you eat in a new way, the world of organic food suddenly becomes very inviting. It tastes better and allows you to feel safe in the knowledge that you're doing the most you can to limit your exposure to the dangers of pesticides, herbicides, hormones, antibiotics, and mercury. Not all food is equally threatening, but within each group there are certainly safer options. Because meat is at the top of the food chain, the toxins stored in its fat are more concentrated and should be your number one concern. Be careful about choosing lean, organic meat, or at least pastured meats (see page 91) if and when you can find them. The same goes for dairy and eggs. This is also the time to make sure you're choosing the purest fruits and vegetables (see pages 94–96 for the best and worst produce). In this section we will also address fish (which cannot be certified as organic and unfortunately contains things like mercury that are harmful to a growing brain) and even plastic water bottles. Drinking enough fluid is essential during these nine months. Though water cannot be organically certified, there are ways to make sure you're getting the purest version possible. We've also included some solid FDA-approved information on other foods that should be avoided when pregnant. The government isn't usually our go-to source for food advice, but when it comes to pregnancy and safety, we feel its guidelines are worthy of consideration, especially with regard to potentially harmful bacteria like *Listeria*.

some basic food risks

Avoiding pesticides, synthetics, and other toxic grimness by eating organic is a great idea. We can't say it enough. But avoiding fertilizer residue won't do you or your baby any good if you don't follow basic food safety guidelines in your kitchen during these nine months. These are good habits to get into. We're talking about avoiding cross-contamination when handling raw meat, washing your hands well and often, and making sure things like dish towels and sponges are completely sanitary. Cook your food well. Use a food thermometer if you're worried things aren't hot enough. Meats should not be consumed raw or underdone (cooking well kills parasites like *Toxoplasma gondii*). Same goes for eggs—no runny yolks for the next nine months. After cooking, refrigerate or freeze leftovers promptly. Wash fruits and vegetables well. Our recommendations are primarily about organics, but germs can be just as harmful to your growing baby.

There are certain bacteria to specifically watch out for when pregnant. *Listeria monocytogenes* can cause an illness called listeriosis, which is particularly dangerous for pregnant women whose immune systems are weaker than usual. It can lead to premature delivery, miscarriage, fetal death, and severe illness or death of a newborn from the infection. If this is enough to make you never want to eat again, don't despair; there are easy precautionary steps to take to prevent it. It may make lunch on the go a bit challenging (see page 127 for lunch advice), but it's obviously worth it.

WASHING AND PEELING

Many people think they don't need to buy organic fruits and vegetables because they peel theirs. This is flawed thinking. Different pesticides have different penetrating qualities, meaning you never really know what crosses the skin and gets into the flesh of a fruit or a vegetable. Peeling isn't enough, and it often takes away important nutrients. The Children's Health Environmental Coalition recommends washing all fruits and vegetables (even organic) before eating to reduce surface traces of chemical residues, wax, and pesticides. If you want to use more than water and a vegetable brush, use plain old mild untoxic soap, not the chemical products marketed to wash fruits and vegetables.

AVOIDING *LISTERIA*

The USDA's Food Safety and Inspection Service (FSIS) and the U.S. Food and Drug Administration (FDA) provide the following advice for pregnant women:

- Do not eat hot dogs, lunch meats, or deli meats unless they are reheated until steaming (165 degrees F).
- Do not eat soft cheeses such as feta, Brie, Camembert, blue-veined cheeses, and Mexican-style cheeses such as queso blanco fresco. Hard pasteurized cheeses, cream cheese, and cottage cheese can all be safely consumed.
- Do not eat refrigerated pâté or meat spreads. Canned or shelf-stable pâté and meat spreads can be eaten.
- Do not eat refrigerated smoked seafood unless it's an ingredient in a cooked dish such as a casserole. This includes salmon, trout, whitefish, cod, tuna, and mackerel, which are most often labeled "nova-style," "lox," "kippered," "smoked," or "jerky." Canned fish such as salmon and tuna or shelf-stable smoked seafood may be safely eaten.
- Do not drink raw (unpasteurized) milk or eat foods that contain unpasteurized milk.

Because *Listeria* can grow at refrigeration temperatures of 40 degrees F or below, the FSIS and FDA advise all consumers to

- Use all perishable items that are precooked or ready-to-eat as soon as possible.
- Clean refrigerators regularly.
- Use a refrigerator thermometer.

another reason to avoid packaged foods

Packaged food containers are sometimes coated with PFCs (perfluorochemicals, the same stuff that's in Teflon) to prevent leaking. If you buy these, take the food out of the box and place it in glass or ceramic jars. Microwave popcorn often comes in PFC-coated bags. Stick to good old-fashioned do-it-yourself popcorn instead.

meat

At this point, your local grocery store is likely to stock some organic chicken, or at least chicken that was produced without hormones and antibiotics. Unfortunately, it's a lot harder to find similar versions of beef, lamb, and pork. This is partially due to the fact that organic feed—what animals need to eat to be certified organic—is expensive. We also suspect that it's because consumers are confused by all of the different gradations of natural meat and don't know enough to ask their butchers to order anything else. "They want you to buy the stuff they're

COOKWARE: YOU CAN JUDGE A PAN BY ITS COVER

Your safest cookware options are cast iron, enamel, glass, and stainless steel. Teflon is obviously convenient, but the chemicals can become airborne and the fumes have been known to kill birds at high temperatures. Also, if you scratch Teflon, the chemicals will get in your food. Cast iron has been known to add iron to your diet—further proof that cooking surfaces do leach directly into your food, which in this case, happily enough, is a good thing.

peddling," says Alice Waters. "If people ask, they will find it." Customer demand is a remarkably powerful thing. What you want to ask for, if possible, is grass-fed, organic meat and organic poultry. The antibiotic-free natural options will suffice in a pinch. We used to have a hard time believing the labels until Marion Nestle, author and professor in the Department of Nutrition, Food Studies, and Public Health at New York University, told us that she assumes even the nonorganic labels are mostly legit. A well-informed skeptic, if she's a believer, so are we.

In our attempt to understand the different designations of meat, we discovered the following extremely helpful definitions and meat certification guide written by the Chefs Collaborative (an organization of food-community members who promote sustainable cuisine and sing the praises of local, seasonal, and artisanal cooking—*www.chefscollaborative.org*).

ALL-NATURAL	The term *natural* may be the most confusing of all. According to the U.S. Department of Agriculture (USDA), a "natural" or "all-natural" label on meat means that it has been "minimally processed and contains no artificial ingredients," yet does not go so far as to prohibit the use of growth-promoting hormones or antibiotics.
GRAIN-FED/CORN-FED	Although there is no official definition, this term describes the usual process of large-scale beef production, during which cattle are fed a diet of "specially formulated feed, based on corn or other grains," according to the USDA. This diet can also include molasses, cottonseed, and protein supplements.
GRASS-FED	According to the American Grassfed Association (AGA) 100% Grassfed Ruminant Program, a grass-fed cow must eat only herbaceous plants and/or mother's milk during its entire life cycle. Grass, the natural diet of cattle, is lower in saturated fats and higher in essential nutrients and creates a healthier, leaner product. To be certified by the AGA, animals must not be administered any antibiotics or hormones during their lifetime. While all beef starts out consuming mother's milk and then grass, most beef is then finished (grown to a desired size and weight) on a diet of grain. Some cattle are fed grass for the last few months of their life to create darker colored meat (see "pasture-finished").

nic pregnancy

PASTURE-FINISHED	These animals receive no grain, nor do they spend time in feedlots or confinement facilities. The AGA, however, distinguishes between grass-fed (never fed a diet of grain, only grass and herbaceous plants) and pasture-finished, which it defines as an animal that has spent a certain amount of time before slaughter eating grass, although it might have eaten a grain diet for most of its life. Some pasture-finished animals eat only organic grass.
ANIMAL BY-PRODUCTS	The USDA banned the use of mammalian bone meal in animal feed in 1997, but still allows such questionable ingredients as chicken feathers, chicken manure, and fish meal to be added to the feed of livestock as protein supplements.
ANTIBIOTICS	Therapeutic antibiotics are used for the treatment of sick or injured animals. Subtherapeutic antibiotics are lower levels of antibiotics than would be used to treat an infection and are used as growth promoters for livestock.
FAMILY VERSUS FACTORY FARMS	The Husbandry Institute, a nonprofit organization dedicated to the humane treatment of animals, defines a family farm as a farm with less than 1,000 animal units, owned and operated by blood-related family members. A factory farm, or large farming operation, is defined by federal and some state statutes as a facility that contains at least 1,000 animal units.

understanding meat certifications

To understand how labels can help you choose the best meat product, read the USDA's organic guidelines (at *www.ams.usda.gov/nop*), which state that in order to be labeled organic, animals must (1) not be fed any rendered animal by-products, (2) must be traced through their life cycle, (3) must not be fed antibiotics or growth hormones and, (4) must be allowed to engage in natural behaviors, such as seasonal access to pasture. These two organizations offer certifications to farmers and companies who go beyond USDA organic standards:

- *Humane Farm Animal Care (HFAC)* is a nonprofit organization created to offer a certification and labeling program for meat, eggs, dairy, and poultry products from animals raised according to HFAC's Animal Care Standards. The Certified Humane, Raised & Handled program HFAC has created has three main points (although the full standards are more detailed and the process is quite rigorous): (1) allowing animals to engage in their natural behaviors; (2) raising animals with sufficient space, shelter, and gentle handling to limit stress; and (3) making sure they have ample fresh water and a healthy diet without added antibiotics or hormones.

• *The Food Alliance* has both fixed standards, which specifically prohibit the use of feed additives or subtherapeutic antibiotics, growth hormones, and genetically modified stock, and scored standards, which focus on more particular practices such as feed production, pasture management, manure management, and animal pest management. The Animal Welfare Institute (AWI) has also set up operational standards called the Humane Husbandry Criteria that farmers who produce meat for companies such as Niman Ranch voluntarily implement in order to receive the AWI certification.

MEAT SURFING: INTERNET SOURCES FOR SAFER CUTS

Heritage Foods USA: *www.heritagefoodsusa.com*
USDA National Organic Program: *www.ams.usda.gov/nop*
American Grassfed Association: *www.americangrassfed.org*
Animal Welfare Institute: *www.awionline.org*
Certified Humane, Raised & Handled: *www.certifiedhumane.org*
Food Alliance: *www.foodalliance.org*
Husbandry Institute: *www.husbandryinstitute.org*
Organic Trade Association: *www.ota.com*
Wild Farm Alliance: *www.wildfarmalliance.org*

Producers and Suppliers
Niman Ranch: *www.nimanranch.com*
Organic Prairie: *www.organicprairie.com*
Thundering Hooves: *www.thunderinghooves.net*

the quest for better meat

Talk to your butcher. If something says grass-fed, you might want to ask how long the animal ate grass—two weeks or six months—before slaughter? You might also want to know how much time the animal you're buying spent out in a pasture versus a confined barn. Don't be surprised if these answers are not on the tip of your butcher's tongue. Consider a new butcher if you don't get the answers you need.

Visit your local farmers' market to find more direct sources to buy meat from. Research local farms online. You may be able to buy directly from a farmer. Think about buying a share of a pig or a lamb with some like-minded friends. Or, if you're a CSA member (see page 18), ask about the possibility of getting weekly meat deliveries. If you can't find meat that satisfies your need on a given evening, turn to other forms of protein like eggs, beans, and nuts (avoiding peanuts). Protein is extremely important to the development of your baby.

fruits and vegetables

We've already preached the gospel of CSA in Part 1, but we can't help mentioning it again. Joining an organic farm is a wonderful, inexpensive way to get produce delivered to your neighborhood and support a small local farmer. That said, growing season isn't year-round in most of the country. Die-hard organic fans forgo eating whatever isn't in season. But most of us have become spoiled by the availability of raspberries in January. When you have to buy outside of your farm and can't find organic, or when you're sitting in a restaurant with no organic options, you should know that not all fruits and vegetables are alike when it comes to pesticide retention.

A 2003 report by the Environmental Working Group (using data from the FDA) found that most of the health risks associated with pesticides are concentrated in a relatively small number of fruits and vegetables, and that people can lower their pesticide exposure by 90 percent by simply avoiding the top twelve most contaminated fruits and vegetables. Over the past six years, the federal government has banned or restricted the use of over a dozen pesticides because of their health risks. Eating the twelve most contaminated fruits and vegetables could expose a person to nearly twenty pesticides per day. Eating the twelve least contaminated will expose a person to only two. Here are a few cheat sheets, with thanks to the Environmental Working Group (*www.ewg.org*):

THE TWELVE MOST CONTAMINATED NONORGANIC FRUITS AND VEGETABLES

(SEE NEXT PAGE FOR BRIEF DEFINITIONS OF CONTAMINANTS)

If you're worried you won't remember everything on these lists, just write down the twelve best and twelve worst on a piece of paper and stick it in your wallet.

FRUITS AND VEGETABLES	MOST COMMON PESTICIDES FOUND	NUTRIENT	SUBSTITUTION (APPROXIMATE NUTRITIONAL EQUIVALENT)
Strawberries	Captan, Iprodione, and Methomyl	Vitamin C	Kiwis, Oranges, Cantaloupe
Peppers (Bell, Green, Red)	Methamidophos, Acephate, and Endosulfan	Vitamins A, C	Green Peas, Broccoli, Romaine Lettuce, Carrots, Brussels Sprouts, Asparagus
Spinach	Permethrin Total and Dimethoate	Vitamins A, C, Folic Acid	Broccoli, Brussels Sprouts, Asparagus, Romaine Lettuce
Cherries (U.S.)	Azinphos Methyl, Myclobutanil, and Carbaryl	Vitamin C	Grapefruit, Cantaloupe, Oranges
Celery	Dicloran, Acephate, and Oxamyl	Carotenoids	Carrots, Broccoli, Radishes, Romaine Lettuce
Apples	Diphenylamine (DPA), Thiabendazole, and Azinphos Methyl	Vitamins A, C, Potassium	Oranges, Bananas, Kiwis, Watermelon, Tangerines
Red Raspberries	Captan, Iprodione, and Vinclozolin	Vitamins A, C	Plums, Oranges, Tangerines
Imported Grapes (Chile)	Captan, Iprodione, and Dimethoate	Vitamin C, Potassium	Grapes (U.S.), in season
Nectarines	Iprodione, Phosmet, and Propargite	Vitamins A, C, Potassium	Bananas, Oranges
Peaches	Iprodione, Azinphos Methyl, and Phosmet	Vitamins A, C, Potassium	Cantaloupe, Tangerines, Grapefruit, Watermelon
Pears	Thiabendazole, Azinphos Methyl, and Diphenylamine (DPA)	Vitamins A, C, Folic Acid	Oranges
Potatoes (U.S.)	Chlorpropham, Thiabendazole, and Endosulfan	Vitamin C, Folic Acid	Sweet Potatoes, Carrots

These didn't make the top twelve, but should be avoided, too: Apricots, Cucumbers, String Beans, Winter Squash.

PESTICIDE DEFINITIONS

For more information about these and other pesticides, go to: *www.pesticideinfo.org* or *www.panna.org*.

Acephate, an organophosphate, is a general-use insecticide.

Azinphos methyl, an organophosphate insecticide, has been singled out for posing high risk to agricultural workers and to the environment.

Captan is a fungicide used to control fungal diseases of turf, fruit, and ornamental crops.

Carbaryl is a common insecticide.

Chlorpropham is a plant-growth regulator used to control weeds in a variety of vegetables.

Dicloran is a fungicide.

Dimethoate is a moderately toxic organophosphate insecticide.

Diphenylamine (DPA) is a crystalline compound used chiefly in the manufacture of dyes.

Endosulfan is a highly toxic chlorinated hydrocarbon insecticide and acaricide.

Iprodione is a fungicide used to control crop disease.

Methamidophos is a restricted-use organophosphate insecticide and an acaracide.

Methomyl, a highly toxic compound in the EPA's toxicity class I, is a restricted insecticide.

Myclobutanil is a common fungicide.

Oxamyl is an acutely toxic insecticide.

Permethrin, an insecticide, is a suspected carcinogen, endocrine toxicant, neurotoxicant, and reproductive toxicant.

Phosmet is an organophosphate pesticide.

Propargite is an acaricide, a pesticide that kills mites and ticks.

Thiabendazole is a preharvest and postharvest fungicide.

Vinclozolin is a fungicide used mainly on vines, fruits, and vegetables.

TWELVE LEAST CONTAMINATED NONORGANIC FRUITS AND VEGETABLES

Asparagus	Cauliflower	Onions
Avocados	Corn (sweet)	Papaya
Bananas	Kiwis	Peas (sweet)
Broccoli	Mangoes	Pineapple

Also relatively uncontaminated: Sweet Potatoes, Plums, Watermelon

dairy

"It's my opinion that if a pregnant woman is going to make one organic choice, that choice should be milk products," says organophile Barbara Kingsolver. "I feel that bovine growth hormones are not something that any developing fetus needs."

Milk is considered the gateway organic food. It's one of the fastest-growing products on the organic market and, at a time when conventional milk sales are dropping, some stores have trouble keeping it on the shelf. It does cost around a dollar more than regular milk, but here's what you avoid by spending the extra money: synthetic growth hormones, pesticides, and antibiotics. As with every segment of the market, there are people who take this a step further and buy local, sometimes not organically certified, milk because they know more about the farms, know the cows are actually grazing on pasture, and prefer to support local farmers. Ronnybrook Farm in upstate New York, for example, has a loyal following. Some local farms won't use growth hormones, but will treat sick animals with antibiotics. However, the amount used is nothing when compared with agribusiness levels.

cheese

Organic cheese is less available than organic milk, even at your local Whole Foods. Persist, though, and you will find. Ask someone at a gourmet cheese store, or go to *www.organicvalley.coop* for suppliers near you. We couldn't have made it nine months without their cheddar to melt, or their butter to spread.

If you can't pass the window of a cheese shop without weeping over a runny Brie, remember you'll be able to have it soon. Meanwhile, there are still other dairy treats you can enjoy, including a wide variety of organic ice creams made by everyone from Ben & Jerry's to Stonyfield. When gobbling these—or even some of the fruit-flavored organic yogurts out there—don't forget to read the labels. Just because they're made with organic ingredients doesn't mean you want food additives or empty sugar calories in your system.

fish

Creatures of the sea present a real conundrum for pregnant women. Fish is so good for you. We read it over and over again in the newspaper's science section. Unfortunately, it is also one of the most contaminated foods out there—the biggest source of exposure to mercury, which can cross the placenta and mess with fetal brain development.

Here's where we normally tell you to buy organic to avoid toxins, but unfortunately there is no such thing as organic fish (yet). The government is in the process of working on a set of criteria for organic aquaculture. And while there are certain farms trying to raise organic fish, without regulations in place, there's no way to know if what you're getting is really organic. Plus, most fish is still wild, making it impossible to certify. And water cannot be certified (something the beauty industry has also grappled with in its quest to create organic certification standards). This means—for the moment, anyway—that even if a fish is labeled organic, it doesn't mean anything. There are a few exceptions to this rule—see our look at one intrepid organic shrimp company on page 102. But until the guidelines are in place, anyone can claim their fish is organic. So don't believe the hype unless you happen to know the farmer and the farming practices. "I'd find a really trustworthy fishmonger and ask them what the practices of the fishermen they deal with are," says Alice Waters. "If they don't know, don't buy the fish there." If you can't find a supplier, Waters says, call up your local organic restaurant and ask them who they buy from. Sometimes suppliers will sell directly to consumers. Fish farms operate similarly to factory meat farms, employing antibiotics, hormones, and genetic modification. Fish can also contain pigment injections to turn their flesh unnatural but more appealing colors. Still, the level of antibiotics and hormones found in farmed fish is much lower than that found in conventional poultry, beef, and pork.

Omega-3s found in fish are important for prenatal and postnatal neurological development. According to the Environmental Defense's Oceans Alive campaign, fish high in omega-3s that are caught or farmed in an ecologically sound manner and are low in contaminants include Atlantic mackerel and herring, sardines, sablefish, anchovies, farmed oysters, and wild salmon from Alaska (fresh, frozen, and canned). Avoid buying farmed salmon; it often contains high concentrations of the contaminants pregnant women should watch out for. This is easier said than done; some stores mislabel and sell "wild" salmon that isn't actually wild. This is another reason to get to know the person selling you your fish. Also, expect to pay extra. Wild salmon will never cost only $6 a pound. If you're interested in fish oil capsules as a source of omega-3s, these can also contain mercury, PCBs, dioxins, and pesticides. Discuss the supplements with your health care provider before taking and purchase only those made from purified fish oil.

All of this begs the question: To eat or not to eat? Some pregnant women just give up fish altogether and get their omega-3s from other sources, like organic eggs and flaxseed oil. Joan Dye Gussow points out that there were landlocked people before all food was transported to and fro who never ate fish and were perfectly healthy; they got the nutrients they needed from other foods. Other women eat the least contaminated fish in moderation. We wish that we could tell you what to do. But as always when things aren't entirely black and white, it's ultimately your choice.

If you choose to eat fish, realize that the more you eat, the more mercury your baby will ingest. And, so far, scientists haven't come up with a how-much-is-too-much figure with regard to fetal brain damage and lowered IQ. It seems like the least harmful way to eat fish, then, is to follow the FDA's suggestions: avoid shark, swordfish, king mackerel, and tilefish. The EPA and some countries, including

Canada and Japan, set their mercury safety standards higher than the FDA. Fresh and frozen tuna should also be avoided. If you're desperate for canned, some states advise eating no more than six ounces a week, while the Environmental Working Group suggests only once a month. Unless you're a total tuna fanatic and have to have it, we say what's wrong with avoiding it for the duration of the pregnancy? There are other fish in the sea.

THE O-FISH-AL LISTS
THE FOLLOWING IS FROM THE ENVIRONMENTAL DEFENSE'S OCEANS ALIVE CAMPAIGN.

CONTAMINATED FISH

How many meals are safe per month? The numbers below indicate the maximum number of meals that can be safely eaten each month. These advisories are for women ages 18–75 based on a body weight of 144 pounds and a meal size of 6 ounces of fish before cooking (if you weigh more or less than that, you may need to adjust the portion size and frequency of eating). For advisories due to mercury, this advice is intended to protect women of childbearing ages and errs on the side of safety for other adults. Fish not on this list are either safe to eat at least once per week, or have not been tested sufficiently for contaminants. For information on fish not on this list, check out *www.oceansalive.org/go/seafood*.

**eco worst, *eco best (these fish are best or worst choices based on the ecological impacts of how they are caught or farmed).

FISH	MEALS PER MONTH	REASON FOR ADVISORY
BLUEFISH	0	PCBs, Mercury, Pesticides
STRIPED BASS (WILD)	0	PCBs, Mercury, Pesticides
AMERICAN EEL	0	PCBs, Mercury, Pesticides
SPOTTED SEATROUT	0	PCBs, Mercury
WEAKFISH	0	PCBs
BLUE MARLIN**	0	Mercury
KING MACKEREL	0	Mercury
SWORDFISH**	0	Mercury
SHARK**	0	Mercury
ATLANTIC SALMON**	½	PCBs, Dioxins, Pesticides

ATLANTIC CROAKER	1	PCBs
WHITE CROAKER	1	PCBs
BLUEFIN TUNA**	1	Mercury
OPAH/MOONFISH	1	Mercury
WHITE MARLIN**	1	Mercury
BLACKBACK/WINTER FLOUNDER	1	PCBs
SUMMER FLOUNDER	1	PCBs
BLUE CRAB	1	PCBs, Mercury
ORANGE ROUGHY**	2	Mercury
SPANISH MACKEREL	2	Mercury
CHILEAN SEABASS**	2	Mercury
WAHOO	2	Mercury
GROUPER**	2	Mercury
EASTERN/AMERICAN OYSTER (WILD)	3	PCBs
ATLANTIC STURGEON**	3	Mercury
STRIPED MARLIN**	3	Mercury
MUTTON SNAPPER**	3	Mercury
ALBACORE TUNA (CANNED WHITE)	3	Mercury
TILEFISH**	3	Mercury
TUNA (FRESH OR FROZEN)	3	Mercury
ROCKFISH (PACIFIC)**	4	Mercury
RED SNAPPER**	4	Mercury
HALIBUT	4	Mercury
MONKFISH**	4	Mercury
BLUE MUSSEL (WILD)	4	PCBs
ENGLISH SOLE	4	PCBs
LINGCOD	4	Mercury

AMERICAN/MAINE LOBSTER	4	Mercury
WINTER SKATE**	4	Mercury
MAHIMAHI/DOLPHINFISH*	4	Mercury
SKIPJACK TUNA	4	Mercury
YELLOWTAIL SNAPPER**	4	Mercury
FLORIDA POMPANO	4	Mercury
BLACK SEA BASS	4	Mercury
DUNGENESS CRAB*	4	Mercury

THE BEST AND WORST FISH

BEST FISH CHOICES		WORST FISH CHOICES	
Abalone (U.S. farmed)	Mussels (farmed)	Caviar (wild)	Salmon—Atlantic (farmed)**
Anchovies*	Oysters* (farmed)	Chilean seabass/ toothfish**	Shark**
Arctic char (farmed)	Sablefish/black cod* (Alaska)	Cod—Atlantic	Shrimp/prawns (imported)
Catfish (U.S. farmed)	Salmon—wild (Alaska), canned, pink/sockeye*	Grouper**	Skate
Caviar (U.S. farmed)	Sardines*	Halibut—Atlantic	Snapper
Clams (farmed)	Scallops—bay (farmed)	Marlin**	Sturgeon (wild)**
Crab—Dungeness, snow (Canada), stone	Shrimp—northern (Canada), Oregon pink, U.S. farmed	Monkfish/goosefish	Swordfish** (imported)
Crawfish (U.S.)	Spot prawns	Orange roughy**	Tilefish**
Halibut—Pacific (Alaska)	Striped bass (farmed)	Rockfish/rock cod** (Pacific)	Tuna—bluefin**
Herring—Atlantic (U.S. Canada)*	Sturgeon (U.S. farmed)		
Mackerel—Atlantic*	Tilapia (U.S.)		
Mahimahi (U.S. Atlantic)			
*indicates fish that are both high in omega-3 fatty acids and low in environmental contaminants		**indicates fish that are high in mercury or PCBs	

anboy farms

...nd an exception to the organic-fish-as-a-marketing-ploy we think is worth mentioning. In 2005, California passed a law banning companies from labeling seafood as organic to protect consumers in the absence of state or federal standards for organic seafood and aquaculture. But there are companies out there trying earnestly to produce the real deal. It helps to be familiar with the good ones, like OceanBoy Farms. Their shrimp is raised in an environmentally friendly way and has been certified organic (according to livestock standards) by a USDA-authorized agency. Their farming operations qualified, as did their plant-processing procedures and their feed diets (the shrimp eat organic feed, which contains no hormones, medications, or preservatives). They use sustainable inland farms and line their ponds to protect the soil. They have mechanized aeration for oxygenation and are secure from disease. OceanBoy still wants the USDA to come up with seafood standards, but, until that happens, their shrimp are sweet and tasty and can be ordered online at *www.oceanboyfarms.com*.

> Pregnant women should only eat seafood that has been properly cooked. Fish should reach 145 degrees F for at least fifteen seconds. Do not eat raw oysters, raw fish, sushi, ceviche, or refrigerated smoked fish.

fishy waters

Don't eat fish caught by friends. Local waters can be highly contaminated even if your friends assure you they know what they're doing. To research local waters: *www.epa.gov/waterscience/fish*. Additional fish resources:

www.checnet.org
www.cspinet.org
www.seafoodwatch.org The Monterey Bay Aquarium is one of the biggest monitors of local waters. Its Web site provides printable pocket-sized seafood guides, regional guides, and solid information on overfishing and sustainability.

what you don't know about bottled water

As we've mentioned, pregnant women need to hydrate. A lot. Unless you have the pleasure of working from home all day long—or in an office with a water filter attached to the tap—you're likely to have to get your H_2O from a cooler in a plastic cup, or, most likely, from plastic bottles.

The jury is still out on the danger of plastic bottles. The American Plastics Council says that they're safe and that public opinion has been swayed by unnecessary confusion about PET bottles. For those of us who don't work in plastics-land, PET (sometimes written as PETE) stands for polyethylene terephthalate, which those in the plastic business refer to as plastic type #1. These letters and numbers can be found inside the ubiquitous recycling triangle stamped on the bottom of all bottles. Different kinds of plastics are labeled with different numbers. (See chart on page 105 for definitions of all seven.) The numbers aren't meant to be read literally, but it's easy to remember that bottles made from PET #1 plastic are intended for single usage. Organically minded people and some scientists are concerned that chemicals in this lightweight, shatter-resistant plastic (used by all companies from Evian to Poland Spring) can leach their way into the water they contain.

Unfortunately, there are no definitive reports on water bottle safety to back up these concerns. One widely quoted study, a master's thesis from a University of Idaho graduate student, argues that toxins from #1 plastics (i.e., water bottle plastic) leach into drinking water. But according to the International Bottled Water Association, the thesis isn't scientifically sound because it wasn't peer reviewed, government reviewed, or published in a scientific or technical journal. The student's project went something like this: 88 percent of bottled water drinkers reuse their #1 bottles for weeks, even months,

TIPS TO MINIMIZE THE USE OF PLASTICS

Use a glass whenever possible. Keep one at your desk at work, or buy water in glass bottles. It's a bit heavier, but worth it.

When you need a portable container, try alternatives to plastics, especially for hot or acidic drinks. Thermoses with stainless steel or ceramic interiors may be too bulky for hiking but are fine for commuting (*www.kleankanteen.com*). Or look into a hiker-style hydro pack.

before recycling them. Over a period of time bottles are subjected to heat, light, and manual pressure, all of which cause the plastic to release unhealthy compounds into the water. Most troubling is a compound called di(2-ethylhexyl) adipate (DEHA), which the student labeled a carcinogen. To avoid DEHA, the study recommends limiting a water bottle's life span to less than a week and keeping it out of the heat and sun.

Given that many plastic #1 bottles are marked with the instructions "Store in a cool, dry, and clean place away from light. Do not refill," the student's recommendation seems reasonable.

While the EPA used to list DEHA as a toxic chemical, for some reason it no longer does. But we're not convinced. We want more concrete evidence that a chemical formerly labeled toxic won't harm us when it leaches out of plastic, especially when we're pregnant or breastfeeding. Exercising caution when it comes to plastic makes even more sense when you take into account another study done by Dr. Patricia Hunt in the April 2003 issue of *Current Biology*, which reported that exposure to bisphenol-A (BPA) causes a chromosomal abnormality in the oocytes, or egg cells, of female mice. Polycarbonate plastic (#7), used for everything from glasses to bowls, is manufactured with bisphenol-A.

In her study, Hunt, a geneticist at Case Western Reserve University in Cleveland, detected a chromosomal error in cell division known as aneuploidy. Other research linked aneuploidy to spontaneous miscarriages and birth defects in humans. It's no surprise that plastics councils here and abroad have disputed Hunt's findings, especially on how they apply to human reproduction or development.

Given all this, we feel safer drinking out of materials that don't break down over time or have the potential to leach chemicals. So we use glass when possible and suggest you do, too. Water from a nonplastic container tastes better anyway. When necessary, we carry wide-necked water bottles

SAFER BETS

When you must use plastics, choose #2 high-density polyethylene (HDPE), #4 low-density polyethylene (LDPE), and #5 polypropylene (PP). These types of plastics are not known to leach harmful chemicals. Avoid #3 polyvinyl chloride (PVC), #6 polystyrene (PS), and #7 polycarbonate. Plastic bottles made from #1 polyethylene terephthalate (PET or PETE) are for single, not multiple, use.

When you do use plastic water bottles made for reuse, store them away from heat. Hand-wash them with a mild detergent and rinse well. Never expose bottles to harsh chemicals, such as bleach, when cleaning.

created for multiple use. And drinking from the occasional plastic #
bottle isn't the end of the world. When we use them, we wholeheartedly r
mend sticking to the master's student's prescription for water bottle safet
go a step further by following plastic manufacturers' own printed-on-the-k
recommendations: only use them once.

	BY THE NUMBERS	
Here's what those numbers and letters surrounded by the chasing-arrows symbol on the bottom of plastic bottles and other food storage containers mean. (If you can't find a number, call the manufacturer directly. On packaged food products, there is usually a toll-free question/comment number listed.)		
Plastic Type	***Used In***	***Our Thoughts***
#1 PET or PETE (polyethylene terephthalate)	Most clear beverage bottles (used by many, including Dasani and Crystal Geyser)	Best used in moderation; recycle after one use.
#2 HDPE (high-density polyethylene)	Opaque food bottles, milk and water jugs	The safest choice if you're using plastic.
#3 PVC (polyvinyl chloride, aka vinyl)	Food containers, some plastic or cling wraps, some soft bottles	Avoid: You know by now how we feel about PVC. Plus some PVC plastics contain softening phthalates (see page 36 for a reminder). If you use plastic wrap, don't let it touch your food.
#4 LDPE (low-density polyethylene)	Used in food storage bags and some soft bottles	A good choice if you're using plastic.
#5 PP (polypropylene)	Used in rigid containers, including some baby bottles and some cups and bowls	A good choice if you're using plastic.
#6 PS (polystyrene)	Styrofoam, used in take-out containers, meat and bakery trays, and, in its hard form, clear take-out containers and some plastic cutlery and cups	Avoid: it leaches chemicals into food, some of which can disrupt normal hormonal functioning.
#7 polycarbonate, or Lexan	Used in 5-gallon water bottles, some baby bottles, and some metal can linings	Avoid: polycarbonate can release bisphenol-A, a suspected hormone disrupter that may cause chromosomal disruption, miscarriages, and birth defects.

There are other things to think about when reaching for a bottle of water. Chemicals are scary, yes. But so are plain old bacteria. In fact, most arguments about the toxicity of water bottles in the media refer to a 2002 University of Calgary study published in *The Canadian Journal of Public Health*. It showed that alarmingly high levels of bacteria (including fecal matter) were in water bottles that were reused without being cleaned. Not surprising when you consider that the bottles were collected from elementary school students who tend not to wash their hands. But it's true that bacteria thrive in warm, moist environments—which is another reason to avoid reuse of #1 PET bottles. If you wash wide-necked bottles specifically made for reuse in hot soapy water between uses (just as you would a glass or a mug) and let them dry thoroughly, they're sanitary.

If you're not convinced plastic is leaching into your bottled water, we have two more thoughts about the bottled water industry that might turn you off it for good. The first is that bottled water isn't necessarily more pure or clean or safe than tap water. In fact, some studies have shown that municipal water (the very thing you think you're avoiding when buying bottled) is actually the source of a significant amount of bottled water sold in this country. It gets processed first and then is sold as purified. The second is political. Some people, such as Marion Nestle, question the entire industry. "I'm stunned by the bottled water scene," says Nestle. "Bottled water has to be the most profitable product ever invented. It's almost impossible to tell what it really costs unless you translate everything into gallons. The bottles come as liters, pints, quarts, and gallons and the prices are impossible to compare. When you do, you find that they range from under a dollar a gallon to more than $100 (at an expensive restaurant). This costs a lot more than gasoline. Clean water should be something widely available to everyone, not just another commodity to buy. Bottled water is undeniably convenient, but much about it is marketing hype to convince you to distrust tap water. If you're worried about water, install a filter. You can carry your home-filtered water around with you and vote with your dollars at the same time."

food storage

You've probably figured out by now that storing food in plastic isn't the greatest idea. Plastic wraps that cling are made from PVC #3, which can leach into your food, especially hot foods or fatty ones like meat or cheese. We realize that everything from sandwiches to vegetables comes wrapped in the stuff, so when you get it home from the store, slice off the layer that was in contact with the offending plastic and re-store it in a ceramic, stoneware, stainless steel, or glass container. It may not be possible to avoid entirely. (For example, we still haven't figured out the best way to repackage meat we're freezing.) If you're carrying lunch to work, these safe containers can be a little heavy. Try wax or parchment paper, one of the new cellulose- or corn-derived "plastics" that have recently entered the market, or cloth bags that can be washed (*www.ecobags.com*). Aluminum foil should be avoided because although it can be recycled, the way it's made isn't earth-friendly. If you're dead set on using plastic storage containers, use only plastics #2, #4, or #5, and no matter what, don't microwave them.

canned goods

Soup is quick, soothing, and easy when you're pregnant and trying to get down all your daily nutrients. Sadly, the lining of most cans contains BPA (bisphenol-A) the suspected hormone disrupter that can also be found in polycarbonate plastic (#7), which leaches into your food. The EPA says the amounts people consume are safe. But when pregnant, we're happy to avoid anything that could mess with the hormones that control fetal development. Many clued-in markets (like Whole Foods) sell beans and tomato sauces in glass jars. Soups and meat or vegetable stocks can often be bought in cardboard cartons. Just don't forget to read the ingredient label!

The Politics of Organics

BY MARION NESTLE

Despite being a longtime analyst of the politics of nutrition, I must confess to a rather late interest in organic foods. Ironically, my epiphany came as a result of an encounter with General Mills, a Minneapolis-based leading global manufacturer and marketer of consumer food products. In 2003, I was invited to give a talk on my book *Food Politics* at a meeting of the Organic Trade Association (OTA) in Texas. With "organic" in the title, I assumed I would be speaking to an audience of counterculture farmers. Wrong. I was introduced by a vice president of General Mills. At that moment, I understood that organic foods are no mere fad; they are big business.

Just how big is a matter of debate. By some estimates organics brought in $20 billion in the United States alone in 2004. Corporations like General Mills know that organics constitute the fastest-growing segment of the food industry. Since 1990, sales have gone up by about 20 percent a year—a gigantic rate by industry standards. Organics may amount to just a tiny fraction of total food sales—estimates range from 1 to 8 percent—but that fraction is rising. Most important of all, Americans are willing to pay more for organic foods. No wonder every big food company wants to get into this business.

To consider organics a passing fancy would be a serious error. Organic farming methods constitute a principled and fundamental critique of the current system of industrial agriculture. This system wastes resources, pollutes the environment, raises animals under unsanitary and inhumane conditions, externalizes every possible cost, and is based on only one rationale—producing the largest amount of food possible at the lowest possible cost, regardless of consequences for health or the environment. At a time when rising rates of obesity are a worldwide public health problem, the accumulation of vast quantities of inexpensive, high-calorie foods may no longer be in any country's best interest.

Certified Organic

The "certified organic" label on a food means that the producers of the food followed these rules: they did not use any synthetic pesticides, herbicides, or fertilizers to grow crops or feed for animals; they did not use crops or feed that had been genetically modified, fertilized with sewage sludge, or irradiated; they did not feed animals the by-products of other animals; they gave animals access to the outdoors and treated them humanely; and they were inspected to make sure they followed the rules in letter and in spirit.

Opponents of organic methods—and there are many—work hard to cast doubts on the reliability of organic certification, to weaken the standards (so there really will be something to doubt), and to make consumers question whether organics are better than industrially grown foods and worth a higher price.

I cannot count the number of times I have been asked whether the "organic seal" really means anything. It does. Ask any organic inspector, produce manager, farmer, or meat, egg, or strawberry producer, and you immediately realize how hard they work to adhere to standards. Trust is essential, and they earn it. As for attempts to weaken the organic standards, think *relentless*. My take: if organic standards require eternal vigilance to protect, they must be good and worth defending.

Given the potential size of the organic market, it is easy to understand why critics are enraged by the idea that producing foods organically might be better for you or the planet. They say that organic methods reduce productivity, are elitist, threaten food security, are an environmental disaster, and are unsafe. Because research on these charges is limited, they are easy to make but hard to refute.

Less Is More

But some questions about organics have been researched and do have clear answers. One is productivity. As early as the mid-1970s, studies questioned the idea that agricultural efficiency depends on inputs of fertilizers and pesticides. In 1981, a careful review of such studies concluded that farmers who converted from conventional to organic methods experienced small declines in yields, but these losses were offset by lower fuel costs and better-conserved soils.

More recent studies confirm these results. Overall, investigations show that organic farms are nearly as productive, leave the soils healthier, and use energy more efficiently than conventional methods. The productivity issue seems settled. Organics do less well, but the difference is small.

If crops are grown without pesticides, you would expect fewer pesticides to get into the environment, foods to contain less of them, and adults and children who eat organic foods to have lower levels of pesticides in their bodies. Research confirms these connections. Pesticides are demonstrably harmful to farm workers and to "nontarget" wildlife, and they accumulate in soils for ages. These are reasons enough to eat less of them. Critics question the safety of organic methods that use manure as fertilizer. But organic standards require farmers to treat manure to make sure harmful microbes are destroyed, and they are inspected to make sure they do so. Growers of conventional vegetables do not have to follow such rules, nor are they held to them. I am aware of only one study that compared levels of microbial contaminants on foods grown organically and not. This found evidence of fecal contaminants on 2 percent of conventionally grown produce, 4 percent of certified organic produce, and 11 percent of produce said to be organic, but not certified. The difference between the first two was not significant. The higher levels on the third suggest that certification means something. I know of no reason why certified organic foods should be less safe, and several why they would be safer.

Better for You?

Do organic methods confer special nutritional benefits? If organic foods are grown on better soils, you would expect them to be more nutritious, and you would be right. This is easily shown for minerals because plants take them up directly from the soil. But plants make their own vitamins and phytonutrients, and those levels depend on genetic strain or treatment postharvest. The idea that organic soils improve nutritional values has much appeal, and organic producers would dearly love to prove it. I cannot think of any reason why organically grown foods would have fewer nutrients than conventionally grown foods, and I have no trouble thinking of several reasons why they might have more, but it is hard to demonstrate that the difference has any measurable effect on health.

Nevertheless, a few intrepid investigators have compared the nutrient content of foods grown organically and conventionally. These show, as expected, that organic foods grown on good soils have more minerals than foods grown on poorer soils. They also show that organic peaches and pears have somewhat higher levels of vitamins C and E, and organic berries and corn have higher levels of protective antioxidants. In general, the studies all point to slightly higher levels of nutrients in organically grown foods. This may be helpful for marketing purposes but is not really the reason why organics are important.

Are foods better if they are organic? Of course they are, but not primarily because of nutrition. Their true value comes from what they do for farm workers in lower pesticide exposure, for soils in enrichment and conservation, for water supplies in less fertilizer runoff, for animals in protection against microbial diseases and mad cow disease, for fish in protection against contamination with organic hydrocarbons, and for other such environmental factors.

My guess is that researchers will eventually be able to prove organic foods marginally more nutritious than those grown conventionally, and such findings might make it easier to sell them. In the meantime, there are plenty of other good reasons to choose organic foods, and I do.

MARION NESTLE is the Paulette Goddard Professor in the Department of Nutrition, Food Studies, and Public Health at New York University and has been a member of the FDA Food Advisory Committee and Science Board. She wrote Food Politics: How the Food Industry Influences Nutrition and Health *(2002) and* What to Eat *(2006). Her diary first appeared in* Global Agenda *magazine.*

CHAPTER EIGHT

home environment

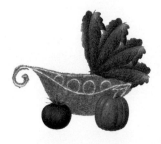

Maybe you're more realistic than we are, but at some point before the pink parallel line popped up on our home pregnancy tests, we indulged in a fantasy or two about how the nine months of pregnancy would be a little like a vacation. If nothing else, we'd get to stop changing the cat litter and pumping gas. So much for fantasy. As you know, there's plenty to get done before bringing home baby. A lot of which involves fixing up your home. We've said it before, but if you take one thing away from this book—and pay attention now—pregnant women should have absolutely nothing to do with the renovation of a home/apartment/garage/garden/office. Erase all those cutesy images of big-bellied women in paint-splattered overalls from the movies, and accept the weird irony that the one time you're finally in the mood to do a little nesting, you will be denied. It's just not safe for you or your baby. If you're joining us late, turn back to Chapter 2 to make sure your house is as safe as it should be. The following section is all about your baby's home environment.

The Precautionary Principle

BY GREGOR BARNUM

My son Sean came into the world in a hard way. Right off the bat he had laryngeal spasms, which completely shut down his respiration. By the time he was two, we didn't know what was going on. We thought he was deaf. I remember one time I stood behind him and slammed a book down on the floor. He didn't flinch.

This was 1984, and we were living in Norwalk, Connecticut. We took Sean down to Seashore, which is UPenn's children's center, and they diagnosed him as autistic. We had been somewhat conscious of a lot of the effects of the environment on what we were creating, but we had no idea that you have to pay attention to things like brand-new carpeting. We went through a major renovation while my former wife was pregnant. There were VOCs in the glues used, new walls, and all kinds of critical chemistries in a number of different cleaning products. I wasn't paying attention, and we didn't restrict the number of chemistries that were intruding into the environment. I don't know how much information was out there, but I know the danger of carpeting had not yet been revealed.

Some people would say Sean's autism is probably genetic, but I would argue with that. There have been ties between autism and vaccinations, but we didn't have Sean vaccinated. Chemical companies rate their chemicals according to how many parts per million are being released into the air, and as long as it falls under whatever part per million, it's considered nontoxic. So even if it's a bad chemical, if it falls under the number, they consider it to be okay. The real question is whether or not these chemicals are accumulating in places that don't have adequate airflow. The other issue is that they're being measured according to a normal adult, and not according to the fragile life systems of a child or pregnant mother. Breast milk is still full of a lot of crap, but I wouldn't advocate not breastfeeding. Breastfeeding delivers antibodies that aren't in formula, and it takes a number of months before enough antibodies collect in a child to allow him to fight for himself.

My grandfather started one of the least environmentally friendly companies on the planet, Rockwell International. It was one of the major defense/space industry builders, and it built airplanes for Vietnam and for most of the Apollo missions. In 1985 the company built nuclear bombs in Utah and was dumping radioactive materials in the salt flats out there. I was a child of the sixties, when it was okay to rage "Fuck you" to the world, but I realized that anger doesn't change anything. So I went to the company, where my family still had people on the board, and tried to explain that it had to clean up their mess.

I learned that there is an ongoing negligence for environmental issues built into corporate America. I began a company that urged corporations to think about not only back-end dumping, but the whole design process. That way, you're building up efficiently while using less of the planet to do so.

We sold the company in '95; it was called RPM systems and it had a similar mission to Seventh Generation, where I now work. The point is to take into account your impact on seven generations out. I started working with Jeffrey Hollender, the president and CEO of Seventh Generation, in the last three years.

I have to say, in the midst of all this, I thank God for Seanie. I would have never understood humanity at this level. But there's still a part of me that feels a certain responsibility at not having paid attention enough.

The precautionary principle (which states that you should avoid the unknown) is something to really pay attention to. I don't want women to walk around feeling paranoid. That's not cool. But you should be able to ask the right question: "Is the environment I'm in right now safe?" I would say pregnant women should not be walking around a new building construction. I would have them read about every piece of whatever-it-is that's going into their house. Anything they're bringing into their house in the terms of outside chemistry—pay attention.

The oddity is, there are no data. There are 90,000 chemicals, and we know only the long-term effects of 3,000 of them. Everyone's saying we're walking experiments because we don't know. It's like, wow.

At Seventh Generation we're always thinking about how to educate people, how to get out there. It's already changing a lot with the rise of Whole Foods and Wild Oats, and smarter consumers. I sometimes think that my generation will die out and the newer generation will be questioning a lot more. As much as we wanted to walk the streets of Washington and change the world, we didn't really think about it. We assume there's a

the nursery

When setting up a nursery, keep in mind that items you might want from small organic stores will take longer than you think to be shipped. Allow plenty of time, or you'll be running through Buy Buy Baby in labor with a plastic changing table in your shopping cart. All the furniture in your nursery, and ideally the entire house, should be made of solid hardwood with a nontoxic finish. Avoid particleboard and plywood, which are held together with toxic formaldehyde-based glues, as well as plastic. We realize that plywood is ubiquitous. If you have something that's made of plywood, you can seal it with Safecoat Safe Seal, a water-based low-gloss sealer for highly porous surfaces. Or speak to a Safecoat salesman about the best product for wood you want to seal.

Our basic advice is that you really won't need half the stuff everyone insists you and your new pumpkin-sized roommate will need. We prefer to spend more money on fewer items. If you're having trouble finding certified or recycled wood furniture for the baby, try to buy secondhand, or inherit hand-me-downs. Americans use about 27 percent of the wood commercially harvested worldwide. Much of it is harvested in an unsustainable (not naturally regenerating) manner, making the burden on forest ecosystems that much greater.

The rest of your baby's environment should conform to the same nontoxic criteria we've laid out for the other parts of the house. If you're worried your baby will scrape her knees learning to crawl on an uncovered wood floor, don't be. The fact is, a bare wood floor is the safest and best possible choice for your home and nursery because it has minimal toxins and can be easily cleaned. According to the CDC, asthma is on a sharp rise in the United States—the number of deaths in children and young adults nearly doubled between 1980 and 1993. The main cause is dust mites, which live in bedding, carpets, couches, and pretty much anywhere there is moisture. Their excrement is a strong allergen that triggers asthma attacks. That said, this is also a bad time to rip up wall-to-wall carpeting, unless you're able to go stay somewhere else for a safe amount of time.

If you're putting rugs down, buy ones made of natural fibers—wool, cotton, hemp. And remember to get a nontoxic skid pad. Also be extra sure any carpeting you do buy doesn't have a backing made of PCB, which is the source of that new-carpet smell. If you have an old carpet, it's probably done off-gassing by now, but make sure to keep it clean. Use the most nontoxic cleaner you can find. If you have a big rug and need to rent a steam cleaner, use less liquid soap than recommended. The water is doing most of the work anyway.

SAFE PAINT

If you're going to paint your nursery, plan on having it done when you can be out of the house for a week (it all depends on the paint, but three weeks would be even better), ventilate extremely well, and be absolutely sure to use a zero-VOC paint with little to no hazardous fumes. The VOC (or volatile organic compound) content is usually listed in grams per liter, ranging from 5 to 200. Even zero-VOC paints have some amount of toxins. Currently the non-milk-based paint we're the happiest with is Safecoat (*www.afmsafecoat.com*). Milk-based paint is just that, and while pure, it's less durable than non-milk-based paint. For more on paint, see pg. 48.

---

sleeping: beds, mattresses, and box springs

Because of a 1973 U.S. law requiring that mattresses meet requirements for cigarette-ignition resistance, it's hard to find a healthy mattress without the fire-retardant chemicals that pose significant health risks. A report by Environment California Research and Policy Center says that some of the most commonly used fire-retardant compounds are PBDEs, which have recently been accumulating in humans, specifically in breast milk. PBDEs are a lot like PCBs, which have been banned for nearly three decades because they cause immune suppression, endocrine disruption, cancer, and behavioral problems. According to the ECRPC report, exposure to PBDEs may be especially harmful to infants and fetuses. In February 2003, the European Union officially banned the use of some varieties of PBDEs in electronics, with more bans anticipated. No such luck stateside. PBDE levels in the breast milk of Americans are reported to be up to sixty-six times higher than in that of Swedes.

It's not a good idea to spend over half your life in a cloud of chemicals. In addition to flame retardants, remember that the cores of many mattresses are made with polyurethane foam, which emits nasty VOCs. To purify your own and your baby's sleeping environments, you will want to purchase an untreated cotton mattress (organic, if you can afford it), a natural latex one, or some combination of the two. Added bonus: organic crib mattresses don't come wrapped in the layer of vinyl that traditional ones do, and they're actually affordable, at about 1/8 the size (and price) of adult mattresses. There's one glitch: the U.S. Consumer Product Safety Commission–required cigarette test. We're not sure why it thinks babies are smoking in bed, but in order to meet these standards, chemical fire retardants are almost impossible to avoid. The alternative versions we mentioned often require a doctor's prescription stating that you or your baby has chemical sensitivities. There are some manufacturers who comply with federal flammability standards by wrapping their flame-retardant-free mattresses in a layer of naturally fireproof wool, bypassing the need for a doctor's prescription. But be sure to find out if the wool is processed with bleaching chemicals.

As for the mattress core, natural latex is the environmentally preferred stuffing, a rubber-tree product that can be sustainably sourced. Some mattresses are stuffed with a mix of natural and synthetic latex, as the latter substance is cheaper (although chemicals are added in the manufacturing process). Both choices are better than the polyurethane foam found in most conventional mattresses. Still other mattress cores have an innerspring system and batting, often cotton. Innerspring mattresses are a popular crib choice; some people think their firmness prevents SIDS.

Once you've answered the mattress question, you'll still have to consider what lies beneath. Many box springs are made of hardwood, but some less expensive box springs are constructed of plywood or particleboard, both of which often contain formaldehyde. Some plywood manufacturers also use pentachlorophenol, a probable human carcinogen, as a preservative. Look for a box spring made from natural, untreated solid wood. Look for "beechwood finishes"; they are among the most natural used.

You'll also need to think about what else you're pressing your body against while you sleep. Invest in an allergen-barrier encasement for your conventional mattress to help keep dust mites away. Dust mites cannot live in organic pure-grow wool mattresses, which is another great reason to invest in one. See www.allergybuyersclubshopping.com for a solid selection, and for a good variety of crib mattresses, try www.egiggle.com. Sheets shouldn't be permanently pressed or made of nylon or synthetic materials. But not just any cotton sheet will necessarily do. A lot of cotton is bleached (sometimes with sodium hypochlorite, which releases dioxin when manufactured) and treated with dyes. Most labels state whether or not they've been treated or are 100 percent natural, but beware. Your safest options generally include simpler solids, neutral colors, and, of course, 100 percent certified organic (pesticide-free) cotton. For more information on organic cotton, see page 150.

$1,500 for a mattress not an option?

Futons are often much cheaper than organic mattresses and box springs. If you decide to get one, try to find a frame made from untreated, certified wood. They're often sold with untreated, organic cotton or wool mattresses, which might require a doctor's prescription. Some natural (nonorganic) futon mattresses are made from green cotton (which is environmentally friendly conventional cotton, harvested without the use of chemicals) and contain nontoxic borate powder as their flame retardant. This is obviously preferable to PBDE. Top-of-the-line organic crib mattresses are less expensive than adult ones. Expect to spend between $250 and $600.

what lies beneath

Sometimes it seems like everyone wants you to put your baby down on plastic. So many things come wrapped in it—from conventional crib mattresses to pack-and-plays to bouncy seats. Our alternative to the ever-present vinyl waterproof pad is to use Pure Grow Wool as a wetness barrier. This wool is made from animals who grazed on pesticide-free pasture and ate chemical-free feed. Puddle pads can be found on many of the sites listed below.

NURSERY SOURCES

A few sites for organic wool and cotton bedding, receiving blankets, bassinets, and co-sleeping accessories, plus cotton and wool futons and mattresses (many of which bear the stamp of approval from nontoxic home goddess Debra Lynn Dadd). For organic cotton clothing and stuffed animal resources plus nontoxic wood toys, check out our organic baby shower resources on page 151.

www.egiggle.com
www.gaiam.com
www.vivetique.com
www.coyuchi.com
www.daxstores.com
www.ecowise.com
www.abundantearth.com
www.shepherdsdream.com
www.babybunz.com
www.heartofvermont.com
www.home-environment.com
www.kushtush.com
www.thenaturalsleepstore.com
www.organiccottonalts.com
www.whitelotus.net
www.greennest.com
www.humanityinfantandherbal.com
www.littlemerryfellows.com
www.theorganicmattressstore.com

CRIB SAFETY STANDARDS

We're all for hand-me-down nursery furniture. Lexy's daughter, Aili, sleeps (whenever she's not in the family bed) in Deirdre's nieces' old crib. Just make sure any crib you're inheriting adheres to the following U.S. Consumer Product Safety Commission standards:

- No more than 2³/₈ inches between crib slats, so that the baby's head and body cannot fit through the slats.
- No missing, loose, broken, or improperly installed screws, brackets, or other hardware on the crib or mattress support.
- A firm, snug-fitting mattress, so the baby cannot get trapped between the mattress and the side of the crib.
- A mattress support that does not easily pull apart from the corner posts (give it a good tug).
- No corner posts over one-sixteenth of an inch above the end panels, so the baby's clothing cannot catch and strangle her.
- No cutout areas on headboard or footboard that could trap the baby's head.
- No splinters or rough edges.
- No cracked or peeling paint.

To be certain the crib remains safe as long as your baby sleeps in it:

- Tighten all nuts, bolts, and screws periodically; check hooks regularly—open hooks may allow mattress to fall.
- Whenever the crib has been moved, make sure all mattress support hangers remain secure.
- Keep the crib at a safe distance from windows, so there's no chance your baby can fall out.
- Make sure there is no drapery or cords hanging within baby's reach.
- Move shelves and tabletops holding lamps, etc., out of potential reach.
- Keep all toys out of the baby's crib or wherever the baby sleeps.

air filters

As a general rule, we don't recommend air filters because the air they produce is never as pure as outdoor air, even in the city. If for some reason you can't ventilate a room, or you've tested and find that, despite your best efforts, pollutants remain, here are some things to consider: First of all, what do you need to filter, and how much money are you willing to spend to get the job done? There are two types of pollutants, particulates (which include dust, mold, pollen, soot, smoke, and dander) and gases (VOCs from paint, plastics, and solvents). Air purifiers can't do much for gaseous pollutants, but they will get rid of particulates, which cause asthma and allergies.

TIPS FOR IMPROVING INDOOR AIR QUALITY
(From the Washington Toxics Coalition: www.watoxics.org)

Source control should always be the first step. Identifying and eliminating the source of specific indoor air pollution is the most effective and long-lasting strategy to improve air quality.

Improving ventilation is also very important. Simply opening windows whenever possible, running window fans or air conditioners, and using exhaust fans in kitchens and bathrooms can help improve indoor air quality.

Air cleaners can also be used, but the above two strategies should be used first. There are various types of air-cleaning devices, and some are more effective at removing certain types of pollutants—such as particulates—than are others. We recommend avoiding "ozone-generating" devices, because ozone—even at relatively low levels—is a dangerous, irritating gas. And because children breathe more air per pound than adults, it could be especially harmful to them. See the links below for information on choosing an air-cleaning device.

- *www.epa.gov/iaq/pubs/insidest.html*
- *www.epa.gov/iedweb00*
- *www.doh.wa.gov/ehp/ts/IAQ*
- *www.lungusa.org*
- *www.epa.gov/iaq/pubs/residair.html*

een house effect

Not only do plants convert carbon dioxide to oxygen, but some remove chemicals, too. All the more reason to thank them every so often. The following list of indoor plants will help filter the air in your home:

- Aloe vera (formaldehyde)
- elephant ear philodendron (formaldehyde)
- English ivy (benzene)
- ficus (formaldehyde)
- golden pothos (carbon monoxide, benzene, formaldehyde)
- peace lily (benzene, trichloroethylene)
- spider plant (carbon monoxide)

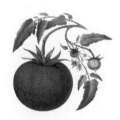

work environment

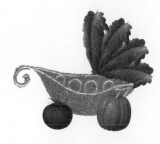

We've talked about what aspects of cubicle life are under your control. Unless you're building your own office, not many. If you are setting up a home office, follow our advice from the Home Environment section and use only nontoxic materials. If you have a printer, scanner, photocopier, or a fax machine, keep things extra well ventilated.

While you might not be telling everyone at work your news just yet, find one trustworthy person to confide in. This can make all the difference if you have to run out of a meeting, or if you need someone to cover for you when you have a lengthy OB appointment. If you feel comfortable enough, try to choose someone in a position of superiority. They can help you change desks without raising any red flags in the event that the office is being painted, or if you happen to sit next to the copier room.

transportation

If you drive to work, you should be aware that, regardless of how clean you keep it, the inside of your car is still one of the most polluted environments in your life. Outdoor pollutants become concentrated in the small space of your car. Keep the window cracked when possible. Do not pump gas when pregnant (or breastfeeding) because gas contains benzene, a known carcinogen, the reproductive effects of which have not yet been proven. Get your partner or a friend to fill you up on weekends. Also, if you're making do with an old car, keep it well tuned, because now is not the time to buy a new one. That new-car smell is a toxic cocktail of off-gassing phthalates and stain-proofers.

If you use public transportation, try whenever possible to sit near an open window. And resist the urge to squeeze antibacterial gel all over your hands after holding a subway pole. Instead, avoid touching your mouth, and wash your hands when you reach your destination.

Mad Scientist

BY ERIKA SCHREDER

For the past ten years, I have worked as a scientist in the field of environmental health, seeking to identify and address factors that can affect our health and the health of our children. My primary focus has been on pesticides—chemicals designed to eliminate insects and other pests. Not surprisingly, a number of pesticides have been found to also harm people, with the potential to cause cancer, birth defects, reduced fertility, and harm to brain development.

The decision several years ago to have my own child brought these concerns into sharp focus. While most women, once they become pregnant, seek to protect their growing child from alcohol, tobacco, and other potentially harmful substances, I was determined to protect my child even before conception.

How? Well, first I cut my husband off of alcohol and caffeine, having read that they posed a potential threat to his fertility. I took some simple steps like making sure my diet was organic and keeping my distance from strong cleaners and solvents. We thought we were ready to go when my husband came home from work one day and told me pesticides had been sprayed inside his office. I did some research and, indeed, the insecticide that had been used is one that has been found to affect hormones.

I guess that was my first moment of maternal anger at someone harming my child—and I wasn't even pregnant yet. My husband had explicitly requested that no pesticides be used, and yet now he had been exposed to a chemical that might affect our ability to conceive or the health of our child. Perhaps most frustrating was knowing that the spray was totally unnecessary, since other, nontoxic methods would provide a more permanent solution.

To be on the safe side, we waited a few months before trying to conceive. I don't really know if we were too cautious, or not cautious enough. Were there still residues at his workplace? How long-lasting could the effects be in his body?

What was even more troubling to me was the growing body of research that this exposure was probably only one of many that could affect our child. I just read of an ongoing study led by scientists at the Harvard School of Public Health that has found connections between phthalates—chemicals commonly used in personal care products and plastics—and reduced sperm volume and quality. I didn't know about this when we were trying to conceive. Should I have been monitoring my husband's aftershave more closely?

I did everything I could think of to protect my child before conception and while I was pregnant, and still do now that she's an energetic and curious preschooler. But the sad truth is that even experts like me can't control all the factors to ensure that the womb is a pure, healthy environment for the child to grow in.

Even though I study toxic chemicals every day, I have many more questions than answers. There are more than 80,000 in use in this country, and less than 5 percent have been tested for their effects on human health and development. In some cases, like lead, it took decades of documenting serious ill effects before it was removed from products like paint and gasoline. Are phthalates the next lead? Or is it going to be one of the hundreds of pesticides for which evidence of harm is mounting? Or is it toxic flame retardants?

My daughter was born healthy and now she's a smart, enthusiastic three-year-old. I am relieved and delighted with her good health, but I'm also fed up. It is not humanly possible, even for a scientific expert like me, to stay on top of all the potential risks and protect my family from them.

It's not fair or realistic to ask people to be experts and to somehow insulate their families from the toxic chemicals in their food, workplaces, food packaging, water bottles, and cosmetics. Clearly, we need to do what we can to protect our families now. But I am also asking these questions: Can't we make cosmetics without chemicals that might harm our babies? Can't we produce food without pesticides that can keep our children from learning at their full potential?

And perhaps most important: when will our state and federal agencies make sure that companies test the chemical ingredients they use and allow only safe ones in everyday products?

I know these things are possible. I read every day about the growing number of farmers who are producing delicious food without pesticides. About cosmetics companies like The Body Shop that are eliminating phthalates and other toxic chemicals from their products, and companies like IKEA and Dell that have removed toxic flame retardants from electronics and furniture.

I wait impatiently for the day when I can keep my family safe without needing to be an expert on the effects of a dizzying array of chemicals. I am certain that we can achieve this and hope to see this day before my daughter decides it's time to become a mother.

ERIKA SCHREDER is staff scientist with the Washington Toxics Coalition, an organization that protects public health and the environment by eliminating toxic pollution.

getting dressed

We know you need to look good at work, even with a bump. But please don't dry-clean your maternity wear, or anything else for that matter. The active ingredient cleaning your clothes is perchloroethylene, a hazardous air pollutant and groundwater contaminant that causes dizziness, nausea, liver problems, and cancer. The solvent is used by about 80 percent of dry cleaners. If your partner needs to dry-clean for work, at least make sure to remove the plastic covering and air the garments out. A lot of clothing labeled "dry-clean" can be washed safely, or look for a professional "wet" cleaner. They use biodegradable soap, steam, and special equipment to get the job done.

The Lunch Hour Dilemma

BY LEXY ZISSU

It's hard to believe there is nothing to eat in Times Square; it's so huge. So many people pass through the area daily. Surely they're hungry and they find things to eat. But when you're pregnant and searching for organic options, it's basically true: there's nothing there.

Honestly, it doesn't matter where you work. Trying to eat lunch when pregnant can feel overwhelming. If you're following government suggestions to avoid deli meats and certain cheeses unless heated to 165 degrees, as well as avoiding too much canned tuna, what are your options, really? Menus are like minefields. An otherwise edible sandwich might contain brie (*Listeria*). Tossed salads (a former staple of mine) don't have any real weight without protein. But these days cold chicken and feta (*Listeria* and possibly *Toxoplasma gondii,* and more *Listeria*) are off-limits. The idea of asking your deli guy to heat a turkey sandwich to 165 degrees doesn't really seem feasible. And the panini melts most lunch places offer these days are warm, but they're certainly not steaming hot. It's enough to make you want to skip lunch, except you're starving and something inside you is kicking for food.

What to do? Open your eyes. Case your work neighborhood for healthy options. And drop the idea that you're going to get completely organic lunches. I used to think all Times Square had to offer was McDonald's and (not very tasty) slices of pizza. But I found several places within a few blocks from my office that offered very edible lunch solutions. A cute—and clean-looking—catering place down the street had fresh, hot meals and lines down the block. It wasn't organic, but when I asked, they said they try to use hormone-free meats. I even happened on a burger place that sold organic beef, antibiotic-free poultry, organic cheese, and organic popcorn with sea salt. The typical health food joint on the corner mainly sold graying kale and grains that sat all day long on steam tables that didn't seem overly sanitary to me. Neither did its smoothie bar. But its daily roster of (sometimes organic) soups—lentil, squash, and split pea—kept me full and satiated during cooler months. And its organic fruit leather and other snacks got me through afternoons where I normally would have been jonesing for a cup of tea. I also kept my list of least contaminated conventional produce in my wallet. Avocados are on there, so I ate them instead of chicken and feta in my tossed salads, and as protein in wheat bread sandwiches.

Mainly I dragged my lunch to work. I say dragged because I brought enough to graze all day long—not a small amount of food. I had plenty of coworkers mock me as I sat, back shoved firmly against my lumbar pillow, and shoveled my home-brought goodies into my mouth. But no matter. The high school shame I used to feel eating an unpopular-looking lunch didn't resurface. My food was part of my mission. And I was happy to know exactly where the stuff came from: piles of fruit, carrots, and celery; hard-boiled eggs; organic yogurts; hummus or cashew butter on wheat bread. (I, with a heavy heart, avoided peanut butter when pregnant after interviewing a well-known food allergist who said moms with things like excema and allergies—I have both—are more likely to have babies with them if they eat peanut butter while pregnant.) I kept dried fruit, cereal, nuts, and granola in my desk at all times. And most days I washed it all down with a glass jar of home-filtered water.

One caveat: The problem with setting yourself up with this much to nosh on is that you never get out of the office. And you're less likely to get up and wash your hands. So I'd force myself to go out and walk around the block for a little air. Movement is key to lessening back pain. When the women in the travel department next to my desk moved their offices and left behind a Pilates ball, I snagged it and forced myself to stretch on it throughout the day. Plus, it doubled as a chair when people came to sit and stare at my food pile. Oh, and if you're thinking coworkers will be shy about taking food from a pregnant woman's mouth, especially if it's organic and strange looking, think again. My nut-and-dried-fruit stash nurtured many more than my growing baby.

CHAPTER NINE

wellness

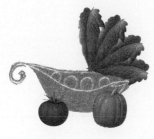

There are a variety of ways to deal with the number of things that will ail you during pregnancy (and which you usually rely on the medicine cabinet to take care of). Below, a collection of all-natural home remedies from friends, many of which were found to be more effective than conventional medication.

heartburn

- Elevate the upper part of your mattress.
- Avoid going to bed right after you eat (particularly if the baby has pushed your stomach up), so the acid from your stomach has less chance to percolate upward.
- Eat an apple every night.
- Eat smaller meals less often.
- Chew your food to within an inch of its life.
- Avoid tomato products.
- Increase milk intake, especially before bed, which might help you to sleep through the night.

headaches

- When headaches start, hop in a very hot shower and stand with your head under the stream until you get some relief.
- ABH—Always be hydrating.

nausea and morning sickness

- Try not to brush your teeth right after you eat.
- Drink ginger, mint, or red raspberry leaf tea.
- Run cold water over your inner wrists.
- Suck on something, anything—a cough drop or a breath mint or an organic lollipop.
- Have your partner rub your feet with lotion before bed.
- Figure out which smells are soothing, and have them on hand.
- Keep something to eat in the morning by your bed so that you can wake up slowly.
- Wear an elastic wristband (sometimes sold as seasickness bands) that has a plastic ball that presses into your inner wrist.
- Carry extra food in your bag at all times.
- Chew on ice.
- Talk to your doctor about taking vitamin B_6. One friend swears it helped decrease vomiting.
- Try acupuncture and/or Chinese herbs.
- Take your prenatal vitamin right before bed to avoid nausea, or try another brand if it doesn't help.

THE DO-IT-YOURSELF ANTINAUSEA WRISTBAND

Take a bracelet-sized piece of inch-wide elastic and fasten with a safety pin so it fits on your wrist (if you're feeling ambitious, sew on a snap). Then sew a round button onto the center of the band. The acupressure point is three-fingers'-width in from the crease of your wrist. If you make a fist you can see two large tendons; the button should land in between them.

RECIPE FOR REAL GINGER ALE

Ginger has long been considered a cure for nausea. We've always loved gi
ale for stomachaches. Here's a more organic version than what comes
corn syrup–filled can:

    2 tablespoons fresh ginger (grated)
    2 lemon rinds
    honey to taste
    1 cup boiling water
    1 quart seltzer

Put the ginger and lemon rinds in a small bowl with the honey. Pour in boiling water
(just enough to cover). Let steep for 5 minutes. Strain and chill. When ready to serve,
add seltzer.

back pain

- Get a prenatal massage.
- Lie on a large inflatable ball and do modified back bends.
- Take a hot shower.
- Use an ice pack or heating pad.
- See a chiropractor or physical therapist.

the waddle

One of our friends is convinced that avoiding "the waddle" for as long as possible
helped immensely in terms of her backaches. Her theory is that the longer you
can avoid giving into the waddle, even if it's temporarily more comfortable, the
better your back will feel in the long run. Stand as erect as possible (instead of
leaning back and letting your belly lead the way) and tuck in your tailbone, which
will put less strain on your back.

sciatica

- Have a prenatal massage if your baby happens to take a nap directly on your sciatic nerve.
- Walk around and do leg squats.
- Take a prenatal yoga class.

constipation

- Talk to your doctor about drinking psyllium in water before dinner every night.
- Take a stool softener.
- Eat dried fruit. Buying organic when it comes to dried fruit is particularly important because the process of drying fruit essentially concentrates any pesticides that are in it.

swelling

- For swollen extremities you might give an herbalist a shot—some of our friends found them helpful.
- Get a foot massage.
- Dip swollen hands in a bowl of ice water.

sleeping

- A full-body pillow for side sleeping can offer relief from aching hips. When placed between your knees, you can also rest your arm on top, which can ease shoulder pressure.
- If the restless center forward's kicking is keeping you awake, moving around can settle her down.

fatigue

- Nap now. It's the last chance for a while.
- Some friends believe in acupuncture; others drink Chinese herbal formulas.
- Even friends who swore off caffeine indulge in a little organic chocolate pick-me-up from time to time.

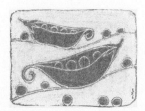

flu shot

If you happen to be pregnant during the fall and winter flu season, your midwife or doctor might suggest a flu shot. The government is all for them, particularly for people with compromised immune systems (and when you're carrying a bundle around, this includes you). The shot given to pregnant women is made from inactivated (dead) viruses (the nasal-spray vaccine, which pregnant women should not take, is made with live viruses), but some women choose to forgo the shot because so many contain the preservative thimerosal (which is made of mercury). Thimerosal has been used since the 1930s to prevent contamination in multidose vials of vaccines. Weigh your options, and make your own decision. Does your job put you at high risk for flu? Flu can be debilitating for the pregnant, lasting much longer than usual. Would you rather have to take fever-reducing drugs and antibiotics later? If you decide to get a shot, ask your doctor to help you track down a preservative-free version. These are single-dose vials that have either no or only a trace amount of thimerosal. Fluzone makes one, so does Fluvirin. Though these mercury-free vaccines are supposed to be reserved for pregnant women and children under the age of two (the population for whom mercury exposure is riskiest), they can be hard to find. You may have to call up various doctors before you hit on one, and then pay out-of-pocket. Vaccination is a controversial subject for pregnant women and parents of young children, but if there's a choice, why not opt for a mercury-free version? For more information on thimerosal and flu shots: *www.cdc.gov/flu.*

ultrasound

Chances are you'll have ample opportunities to see your baby during your forty-week gestation. If your health care provider is an obstetrician, you may be expected to have at least a half a dozen ultrasounds. Midwives tend to perform them less frequently. Women interested in natural childbirth are becoming increasingly skeptical of the technology. There is some anecdotal debate about their safety. Some believe that the sound waves can affect a growing fetus. The medical community dismisses this notion. Some women compromise by trying to have no more than the essential ultrasounds throughout their entire pregnancy. Whatever you choose to do, it might be helpful to know that most moms-to-be do not forgo the benchmark twenty-week fetal anatomical ultrasound.

fitness

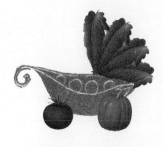

At this point in your life, you've probably figured out a workout you're happy with. Or maybe you started one before you found out you were pregnant. Or maybe you've taken up something as simple as walking. Any which way, we want to encourage you to continue doing what you're doing. If you want to start something new, or get some advice on exercises that might be particularly helpful to you in your new state (in general, you want to be doing ab strengtheners, back strengtheners, and leg exercises), now might be a good time to splurge on a personal trainer. Or get your care provider to write you a physical-therapy prescription and have your health care company foot the bill. However you manage to do it, make sure you move around. Because even when you're exhausted and/or feeling sick, the adrenaline and other hormones that get released from exerting yourself (even a little bit) will make you feel better and sleep better. And a stronger you will mean less back pain and other pain as you get bigger. And bigger. And—did we mention?— bigger.

I'm Not Fat, I'm Pregnant

BY JULIE KLAM

Before I got pregnant, my sister-in-law/pregnancy-marriage guru told me how much pregnancy books frightened her. So when I got pregnant, I stayed away from the books. Except one. A children's pop-up book called *Before You Were Born,* with cute pastel illustrations and rhymes about what happens every month. That, I decided, with my common sense, was enough.

I was always a healthy, organic eater and big exerciser—two hours every other day of cardio. I knew the little pregnancy rules about staying away from tuna and deli meats and cheeses from distant lands and artificial sweeteners. Once, I had a piece of gum in my mouth and when I realized it was sugar-free, I just let it go tumbling onto a New York City sidewalk. Because I was so scared of what that artificial sweetener would do to my baby, I littered! I had aches and pains that I wouldn't treat with ibuprofen and insomnia that I suffered through without drugs. People chirped that it was good practice for when the baby came (a lie, by the way; lying awake at night tossing and turning is not the same as being woken up out of a sound sleep by a infant singing the opening bars of Led Zeppelin's "Immigrant Song"). But the one thing that got the better of me was horrendous, diabolical nausea. Unfortunately, the only cure for me was massive amounts of breakfast carbs—pancakes, muffins, waffles, bagels, whatever. I decided to listen to my body even if it yelled *"Danish,"* and by the end of my first trimester I had porked up twenty-five pounds. I boasted to everyone that it was really a triumph; I had achieved what it took most gals ten months to do in a mere three. I was done. I'd gained all of my weight; the rest of the pregnancy, I could kick back and relax.

But my weight continued to go up, so I checked the pop-up book and saw that at four months, the cute cartoon lady had "gotten her energy back" and was in an aerobics class doing leg lifts. I spoke to my doctor about what I could do for fitness, and she said anything but crunches. I had been in great shape before the pregnancy, but four months of doing nothing but lifting cakelike items to my mouth had slowed me down. I always loved working out, but I dreaded it now, mainly because I looked fat, not pregnant. I didn't know this until I was pregnant, but apparently I have a tipped uterus, so my OB said my belly wouldn't "pop out" till much later. I thought perhaps it was tipped back so far that the baby was actually in my ass, which was expanding at a rate equal only to the Hadassah-lady briskets on the backs of my arms.

It was around this point in my pregnancy when I started to consider the fact there was an "after" looming, and it wasn't going to look good. The baby would be born, and I wouldn't be pregnant anymore. I didn't start to diet, but I knew I had to move, so I really committed to the gym. I loved the feeling I had there—I felt like I was me again, blood moving, endorphins pumping—but hear this: It Had Zero Effect On My Weight. I continued to balloon. The RN at my doctor's office recommended I eat more "chicken and fish and veggies"—instead of carbs. How stupid is that? Has anyone ever thought, "I'd like this slice of babka, but an apple will do the trick"? (I ended up changing my starting weight in my pregnancy chart the next time I was left alone with a pen in the examining room, and was not bothered again by her.) But I was bothered nonetheless. I saw people in my neighborhood walking around with new babies looking svelte and small. Maybe I was carrying one of those *Weekly World News* fifty-pound babies. I could hope. On the elliptical machine at the gym, I watched endless hours of daytime-TV makeover shows in which they taught women who never lost the baby weight how to wear drapey clothes to appear more slender. I began to vacillate between fears of being a bad mother and fears of being a fat mother. By month 8, I was up forty-five pounds. I had a long road ahead, and my hunger was not decreasing.

One hellish August day en route to the gym in week 32, I thought I felt the baby stop moving, so I jumped into a cab and went to the hospital. The baby appeared to be fine, but I was seriously ill with extremely high blood pressure. It was eventually diagnosed as preeclampsia, a condition involving high blood pressure, swelling due to fluid retention, and abnormal kidney function requiring, among other things, bed rest. Good-bye, gym; good-bye, walking the dog. I began "spilling protein"—losing protein in my blood—so the baby wasn't getting the nutrients she needed. The only cure for preeclampsia is delivery, so I went in at thirty-five weeks. The preeclampsia had added around twenty pounds because of the fluid retention, bringing my weight-gain grand total to sixty-three pounds. My early delivery brought me one small bummer; the baby was only four pounds (when she came out, the doctor said, "Ohhh, scrawny!"). I looked exactly the same after she was delivered as I did before, except worse.

In the first two weeks postpartum I lost the twenty pounds from the preeclampsia, and my blood pressure returned to normal. I was far less concerned about my looks than I predicted. For one thing, I couldn't take my eyes off my sweet little Violet, and in the process of putting weight on my preemie, I lost the weight I had gained carrying her. By her first birthday I was back in my old skinny jeans. And Violet, who was born so small she was not on the charts, was now off the charts in size and turning into a gorgeous, kick-ass kid.

As my husband and I contemplate the next pregnancy, I have complete dread about trading my size 0 jeans for the XXL drawstring pajama bottoms. I tell my husband if we were sea horses, he'd have to carry the pregnancy. Next life, he promises. Getting fat and unfat was a drag, but in the scope of things, a really small deal. Obviously, next time I will try not to gain so much weight. I will try not to have such an intimate relationship with the fellas at the bakery counter. But if I do gain weight, I am not beating myself up about it. It's about the baby after all.

It's a very strange thing to live your whole life taking care of yourself and then suddenly become responsible for this entire other human being. They don't do anything without you. You will never come home and get a note from your newborn that says, "Went to the movies, be back soon!" They are totally dependent on you, and that's kind of terrifying, because if you're like me, you used all of the time you had before the baby came quite nicely. And you will have less of this—actually none of this to begin with. But then it changes. Little by little you will find yourself again; your sense of humor, your creativity, your ability to remember what you walked into a room for, and ultimately, even your body. But it will be even better, because it did this amazing thing.

JULIE KLAM is an Emmy-nominated freelance writer who lives in New York City with her husband, daughter, and dog.

the first trimester

This may be a period of time when you don't feel like moving at all. Even if you're not puking, movement can make you feel seasick. Cut yourself some slack. Don't beat yourself up about skipping your workout. But whenever you do feel up to it—even for a brief moment—take a walk, a yoga class, or a (stationary, if your balance is off) bike ride. You'll thank yourself. Just keep in mind that whatever exercise you do now isn't about getting to new levels of strength or stamina, it's about maintenance and getting your blood flowing. If you're having a totally normal pregnancy and are feeling okay, you can continue your regular routine—weights and all—as long as it's comfortable. But back off if you're not. And drop the more jarring parts of your routine, even at this early phase. Jogging may be suitable for someone who has been doing it for years, but sprinting is too strenuous. Same goes for really intense yoga. Certain poses are fine if you're used to them and good at them, but the more high-impact moves should be left behind for now.

When you feel up to it, check in with a professional who has prenatal knowledge. He or she can help you custom design a routine and answer any questions you might have about what you can and can't do. If you have a yoga class you frequent but aren't yet telling people you're pregnant, you might choose to make an exception and share your news with the teacher. He or she might be a great source of important information, especially now that you have relaxin running willy-nilly through your body. This is a hormone released into your system to help you be more flexible months from now during labor. Though it's basically meant to help open up your pelvis for birth, it spreads everywhere. So you have to be careful about not pushing yourself as far as you used to; overstretching is really easy. You may also find that not only are your joints looser, but your balance will start to falter. Certain exercises should be done with a wall or a chair close by for stability.

The first trimester is also a good time to try working out with a heart monitor. At the very least make sure you can comfortably talk to someone when you're doing cardio. If you can't, you're overdoing it. Most important, listen to your body. If you're tired, give yourself permission to stop what you're doing. If you lose a little muscle, so be it. You'll have time in the second trimester and the beginning of the third to gain some of it back. And soon enough you'll have baby-carrying arms anyway.

Meanwhile, it's never too early to think about posture and alignment. Tuck your tailbone in now so you'll be used to it when your belly starts to pull you forward and create an arch. And try not to cross your legs; an uneven pelvis can lead to back pain later on.

the second trimester

Some people say they get an energy boost during these three months. If you're one of these lucky ones, work it while you can. Vary your routine—walk, do resistance, stretch, take a class. Just work out on the days you have the energy. But don't increase the intensity of a workout just because you slept through one or two. You could wind up overdoing it. After twenty weeks most doctors recommend you don't lie flat on your back for any extended period of time. The weight of the baby can press on a vein (the vena cava) that carries blood from your lower body to your heart. The bigger you get, the easier this position is to avoid; it starts to get uncomfortable after a while. So a lot of exercises—from balance ball sit-ups to certain yoga poses—aren't really something you can do anymore. If you're working with a trainer or a teacher, he or she can instruct you on what is available to you now. Or just modify accordingly.

Some of the aches and pains you'll experience in your third trimester will make their appearances now. These include round ligament pains. These ligaments support your uterus. The pains can be quite sharp and scary when they first happen, but they're normal and nothing to worry about. Sometimes you can feel them when you sneeze, or when you move too quickly (like when you stand up from a forward bend in the beginning of a yoga class and aren't warmed up yet). Some women like to rest until the pain subsides; others say it helps to keep moving. Either way, the pain will dissipate and you'll know better to slow it down the next time around.

Keep On Moving

BY KIMBERLY BROWN

After my doctor confirmed that I was pregnant, she cautioned me to take it easy. I'd had a miscarriage about a year earlier and she wanted me to treat the first trimester gingerly. It was not a good time to start a new exercise routine, she warned.

What could be better than doctor-sanctioned laziness? I thought.

During those first hold-your-breath months, I almost pretended I wasn't pregnant. I was petrified of getting attached to a pregnancy that might not stick. So I didn't alter my routine much. I ate decently, maybe tried to eat more protein and vegetables and less junk, and stayed away from the trifecta of prenatal no-no's: fish, booze, and soft cheeses. And I remained pretty sedentary.

But once into my second trimester and having "passed" the fancy ultrasound test that assured me I was at low risk of having a baby with Down syndrome or other major fetal abnormalities, I had to confront the reality that a baby, a human being, was actually growing inside me. I felt an awesome responsibility to do right by her. For me, that meant not only paying more attention to what I put into my body, but, for once, taking good care of myself in other ways.

It was one thing, when operating solo, to cavalierly ignore science, and lots and lots of received wisdom about the importance of exercise to my health and to my figure. But add the little peanut—or, as ours appeared in the ultrasound, the wide-mouthed bass—into the picture, and the stark reality was that I was eating, sleeping, thinking, and *not* exercising, for two. In other words, I'd arrived at that place where health interests, vanity, and my natural tendency to wallow in guilt and anxiety converged. There was only one road out: I needed to start exercising.

I hate gyms. I've never walked into one that didn't make me cringe at its particular scent of drying perspiration. I've invented yeast infections to get out of taking bike rides with my husband. And running makes me feel like my brains are jiggling around in my head. One good friend boxed throughout her pregnancy—no joke—and offered to bring me to her celeb-soaked Los Angeles boxing ring to show me the ropes. But punching people for fun seemed karmically sketchy. After all, I at least had some vague idea that I was growing someone inside of me who I hoped would be a calm and peaceful soul.

Yoga, at the suggestion of my doctor, seemed like the best bet. At least my body would only have to come in contact with the freshly laundered mat I could bring from home.

My experience with yoga before this point was limited, intermittent, and ambivalent. It took years after most of my friends were practicing for me to even try it—just the idea of being that still, and that quiet with myself, would make me squirm.

Once I gave it a chance, I found I actually enjoyed parts of the experience: the smoky incense, the woozy music, and the relaxation and cool-down period at the end. I also liked how I felt after class or after practicing at home with a video. But I never became a regular.

In my fourth month of pregnancy, I started a prenatal yoga class that I chose specifically because it was not held at the famed studio where Madonna practiced while pregnant (before she switched to her Jewish gurus). My spot had no starlets, no pizzazz, and no competitive one-upsmomship. Just low lights, sparkling-clean floors, and the lovely instructor, Siddiqa. A young mother herself, Siddiqa reminded the mothers-to-be to be present in our pregnancies and to try to honor whatever was going on in our bodies and our minds. She reminded us to listen to ourselves and to remember how hard our bodies were working to grow the little beings inside us.

I tried to quash the urge to giggle at her suggestion that my baby could not only hear, but understand every word I spoke while she was in the womb, and that I might want to stop cursing right away. The baby could even absorb my thoughts, she warned. Nevertheless, I worked to give myself over to the experience of mindful meditation, and learning to breathe and focus the "third eye," or what I understood to be my mental and emotional center.

It was thrilling to be able to make some of the stress I'd been carrying around disappear (if only for moments before Siddiqa would kick my ass with partner squats). Or to completely let go, with long sessions of intense free dance. She always brought us back around to relaxation at the end, guiding us into that blissful almost-sleep at the end of class.

My attendance at the yoga classes dropped off when a new job began to occupy my days. But I brought what I could remember into my bedroom over the next several months, practicing on my bed or on the floor, sometimes alone, sometimes with my husband watching or reading nearby, waiting for me to finish so we could have our own little nightly relaxation ritual. Just before we went to sleep, he would apply honey-scented belly butter to my growing middle, a vain but utterly soothing attempt at preventing stretch marks.

Birthing classes soon supplanted yoga as my after-work priority. We came to our decision to try to have a Bradley birth circuitously, after another birthing class didn't work out. (The instructor's home reeked of wet dog and I collapsed into an allergic coughing fit during a meditation exercise on the first night of class.) The Bradley class was the only one we could find that was both highly recommended and possible to complete before my due date.

The more I learned, the more I wanted to have a birth without drugs, to at least try to do what women have been doing forever without medical intervention. The class, which met once a week for eight weeks, was ambitious. It was difficult to complete all the reading. I was often too tired after work to pay close attention in class. But the homework exercises meshed seamlessly with the yoga I already had learned and was practicing at home more and more.

Medical evidence to the contrary, I was terrified that I'd have a breech baby like my sister's first. Midwives teach a modified yoga cat/cow move to help maximize a baby's chance of turning in utero into the head-down position. So even after my baby was beyond the point where there was much chance of her moving out of her perfect fetal pose, each night I would get on all fours, sink my pelvis down and then pull it back up, down and up, over and over and over again, out of total fear of a last-minute flip-flop.

I roped my husband into the partner squats Siddiqa taught me. I tried to teach him how to do squats with the birthing ball too, and together we worked on breathing and progressive relaxation exercises. But I never really saw these exercises as real yoga practice. This really was practice for having a baby.

The day I eased into labor, my contractions began light and irregular. I'd been having Braxton-Hicks contractions for months and these were only incrementally stronger. A call to my doula told me that I was in false labor, which could last as long as a week. So I tried to consider the intermittent pains as trial runs. I would simply breathe through them, and, if need be, use some of the positions I'd learned in class.

But as the day stretched out, and the intensity deepened to the point where I had to pull my car over to the side of the road to sit out the pains, I began to draw more closely on the breathing meditations I'd learned in yoga class.

Sitting in a Thai restaurant the night before my baby was born, I can remember taking a bite of spicy curry chicken and then excusing myself from the conversation with my parents and husband to turn inward, focus on that inner eye, and breathe into my center. There's a picture of me emerging from one of these contractions looking totally at peace.

The Bradley class was great instruction in what to expect during delivery, and tools for getting through with the help of a birth coach. But without learning how to breathe in yoga class, without the practice of listening to myself and to my body, I could not have had a drug-free delivery.

Immediately afterward, my doula and my doctor were telling me what a rock star I was for making it through without any drugs. (At our hospital, 98 percent of the vaginal births are said to involve epidurals.) So their praise felt great, but I swore then that I would not endure another labor without drugs.

Now, four months later, I'm pretty sure that if I get pregnant again, I will try for another drug-free delivery. Natasha arrived alert, she suckled immediately, and my recovery was shockingly easy. I'm convinced that not having drugs had a lot to do with that. And I'm certain that without having learned, through yoga, how to inhabit my body—to listen to it and honor it—I would not have had the birth I wanted.

I'm still continually in awe of our daughter, and of the fact that she came from my body and is completely nourished by it. I have so much new respect for what I can do. For what my body can do. And I plan to teach Natasha how to respect, cherish, and use her body well.

She will grow up with a mother who doesn't need or want a doctor's excuse to be lazy.

KIMBERLY BROWN is a journalist living in Los Angeles with her husband and their daughter.

the third trimester

Continue to work out however you can, paying careful attention to alignment, posture, and balance. When you wake up feeling like a creaky old lady, it's amazing how twenty minutes on a stationary bike can de-creak you. Ditto a few arm stretches. At the very end you may find yourself slowing down. Let it happen. Your body has managed to grow this baby on its own, it knows what it needs. Expect to lessen the amount of weight you lift and the degree of difficulty. If you can't do anything else, walk.

If getting to a gym is too much trouble, have a few things on hand at home—a balance ball, a mat, some resistance bands or tubing—that can keep you moving around in your own surroundings. Just don't start anything new or strenuous at this stage of your pregnancy without consulting with an expert. Here are some suggestions on how to cope with third-trimester body demons.

feet and ankle issues

Water retention and loosening ligaments can make your feet stretch, ache, and even grow. It can sometimes feel like bones are about to poke through your heels from the extra weight you're hauling around. Try flexing and pointing your feet and rotating your ankles throughout the day. Soak swollen feet in cool water. Wear cotton socks so your skin can breathe. And make sure your shoes are padded enough. Consider going up a half size if they're feeling tight. Elevate your feet as much and as often as possible.

lower back pain

Strong lower abs will help with lower back pain. So will good posture. A physical therapist can help check out your alignment and show you how best to sit at a computer desk all day long without exacerbating back pain. Look into buying a lumbar pillow. Get up and stretch whenever you feel the need.

leg cramps

Sometimes these cramps are due to dehydration. Make sure you're drinking enough water. To improve circulation, try support stockings. Elevate legs whenever possible, and try not to stand around for too long. If you get a cramp, pull your toes back in order to release it.

shoulder pain

Women start sleeping on their sides when they're no longer supposed to sleep on their backs (the middle of the second trimester). This can lead to crunched shoulders. Large maternity pillows sometimes help. So do extra pillows in general.

managing aches and pains

The aches, slight pulls, and general soreness you might formerly have cured with ibuprofen are a daily fact of pregnant life. Ibuprofen shouldn't be. Doctors and midwives say Tylenol is okay to use if you really need it. Luckily, ice, heating pads, and warm baths (nothing hot enough to raise your temperature) often do

OM SHANTI

With all of our talk about toxic plastic, we'd be remiss not to mention the obvious: most yoga mats are synthetic, plastic, and often include PVC. Luckily there are plenty of (machine-washable) organic alternatives. A quick Google search will offer a large variety, from hemp to organic cotton to open-cell natural rubber (which is a bit stinky, frankly). Be warned: these are often bigger, clunkier, and less portable than regular synthetic yoga mats.

the trick nonmedically. Acupuncture and massage can also help with more intense pain. If you don't have the time or money to spend on seeking help outside your home, ask your partner to rub out your kinks with oil. A good organic oil will do, maybe even one with arnica in it, which naturally does what Ben-Gay does. Olive oil is a good in-house option. If you're past being able to lie on your stomach, sit backward on a comfortable chair, leaning on a pillow. Or lie on your side and prop pillows between your legs. Both positions will afford your partner easy access to your back. If and when your lower back and butt start to get sore from toting around extra weight, an at-home massage by your partner is a must. It's hard to ask a masseuse to really rub your butt the way you need it rubbed!

GOLF

It may seem, especially to fans, that pregnancy would be a great time to hit the links. You get to walk around, move your arms, sit in the cart if you get tired. Plus all that fresh air, right? Well, maybe. There is no telling how many pesticides, herbicides, and rodent killers (remember *Caddyshack*?) are used on any given course. *Home Safe Home* author Debra Lynn Dadd found that pesticides are applied to golf courses at higher concentrations per acre than almost any other type of land, including farms. Ask the management, and depending on what you hear, be prepared to stash your clubs for a while.

play

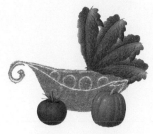

On the days you're feeling good, get out there and enjoy yourself. A few assorted precautions to keep in mind before you start gardening, playing with your pets, or planning a baby shower.

gardening

What feels more back to nature than working in the garden? Nothing, as long as you have switched to nontoxic insecticides, plant foods, and weed killers. You'll have to pay more attention than you think necessary at your nursery. Ask questions about every product you use. And never forget your trusty gloves when handling soil. *Toxoplasma gondii* is an unsafe parasite that causes an illness called toxoplasmosis, which nonpregnant people can handle, but which can be extremely threatening to a fetus. The parasite can be found in soil (as well as in the litter) if your cat has eaten any rodents or birds. Cats often use gardens as their outdoor litter boxes. If you employ a lawn care service, find out what products they use. If you're not satisfied with the answer, finding a more organic service will provide you with the peace of mind you're looking for. For more information, see *www.organicgardening.com* or *Organic Gardening*, by Maria Rodale.

pets

Besides being a source of guilt in the months leading up to the birth of your new and improved love object, pets can also be toxic. Most flea baths, collars, bombs, and shampoos are not things you want on your skin or in your lungs. Opt for more organic versions. Now is also not the right time to get a new cat. If you do, have the animal tested for toxoplasmosis before she enters your home (and heart).

cat litter

If you've ever changed a litter box, you're all too familiar with the dusty cloud that wafts up as your pour the granules into the (inevitably) plastic box. Most litters are clay. The fancier clumping litters are made with sodium bentonite, a naturally swelling clay. The dust from both contains crystalline silica, a carcinogen. Couple that with the fact that most litters contain added fragrance to mask odor, and you know that dust cloud is not something you want to be breathing—even if you're not changing the cat litter to avoid toxoplasmosis—when pregnant. Plus, clay isn't biodegradable and clumping clay can be very dangerous for your kitty when ingested. Greener litter options are available, made from corn, wheat, alfalfa, wood, and newspaper. They have their pros and cons. These litters are, unlike clay, biodegradable and flushable. If you can't find them at a local pet store, they're widely available online. But many feline owners complain they don't work anywhere near as well as clay. Try them and decide for yourself.

organic baby shower

As soon as people realize you're pregnant, there's a good chance they're going to start slipping you gifts to celebrate. It's a really lovely acknowledgment of what's to come. Unfortunately, they'll include a lot of phthalate-filled plastic toys and vinyl books. It may sound harsh, but when possible, sneak these back and exchange them for more natural versions. (Your child will start sucking on paper books bleached with chlorine soon enough.)

When it comes time for a baby shower, take some control and apply our less-is-more rule. Tell whoever is organizing it to spread the word that you'd be much happier with fewer organic items versus a nursery of plastic. You could register at an organic store or possibly even include a list of Web sites (see page 151) in the invitation.

organic cotton baby clothing

Ideally your baby's wardrobe will be hand-me-downs (preferably from someone with good taste!). This is a great way to recycle. There isn't much point in buying everything new; babies grow so fast, sometimes they don't even make it into the outfits you carefully purchased. No matter how many T-shirts with whimsical sayings you already have, or pink-patterned onesies you don't need, friends and family will inevitably give you clothing as gifts. There's just something irresistible about baby clothes. If you register for baby gifts, or are buying new, seek out organic cotton, which is grown the same way organic food is. According to the Sustainable Cotton Project, each T-shirt made from 100 percent organic cotton keeps one-third of a pound of synthetic fertilizers and farm chemicals out of the environment. If you can't find organic cotton, the next best thing for your baby is 100 percent cotton. What you want to avoid are fabrics like flame retardant–treated nylon and polyester, which don't allow a baby's skin to breathe and can cause rashes, to say nothing of what those small lungs might be inhaling. Federal flammability standards require children's sleepwear to be flame-resistant, and if the fabric ignites, the flame must self-extinguish. But snug-fitting sleepwear made of stretchy cotton meets the same safety standards as synthetic fabrics. If it fits closely enough against a baby's body, and has no air underneath it to feed a fire, it won't ignite or burn rapidly.

MORE REASONS TO BUY ORGANIC COTTON
(From the Sustainable Cotton Project)

- Cotton uses about 25 percent of the world's insecticides and more than 10 percent of the pesticides (including insecticides, fungicides, miticides, herbicides, defoliants, and growth regulators).
- In the United States, 25 percent of all pesticides used are applied to cotton.
- In California, five of the top nine pesticides used on cotton are cancer-causing chemicals (cyanazine, dicofol, naled, propargite, and trifluralin).
- All of the top nine cotton pesticides in California are labeled by the U.S. Environmental Protection Agency as Category I or Category II materials, the most toxic classifications.
- In India, 91 percent of male cotton farm workers regularly exposed to pesticides eight hours or more per day experience some type of health disorder, including chromosomal aberrations, cell death, and cell decay.
- Cotton fibers account for almost 50 percent of the textile market worldwide.
- Globally, nearly 90 million acres of cotton are grown in more than seventy countries. The United States is the second-largest cotton producer in the world, growing approximately 19 million bales worth $6 billion in 1997 (enough to make approximately 9,215,000,000 T-shirts).
- As much as two-thirds of a cotton crop can creep into the food chain. Each year, half a million tons of cottonseed oil make its way into salad dressings, baked goods, and snack food; another 3 million tons of raw cottonseed are fed to beef and dairy cattle.

For more information check out *www.sustainablecotton.org*.

wish list

Here are a few sites we wish anyone buying a baby present for us would surf. Some sell (adorable) clothes and baby blankets; others stock toys not made of plastic. Many of the nursery resources listed (page 119) also sell sheets, blankets, and baby clothes. If you don't need any more stuff, ask for a subscription to your parenting magazine of choice or our trusty resource, *The Green Guide.*

Under the Nile: *www.underthenile.com*
Bamboosa: *www.bamboosa.com*
Sage Creek: *www.sagecreeknaturals.com*
Organic Gift Shop: *www.organicgiftshop.com*
Organic Selections: *www.organicselections.com*
Organic Wear USA: *www.organicwearusa.com*
Our Green House: *www.ourgreenhouse.com*
IIKH: *www.twokh.com*
Crystal Baby Organics: *www.crystalbabyorganics.com*
Danish Woolen Delight: *www.danishwool.com*
Island Treasure Toys: *www.islandtreasuretoys.com*
Om Bebe: *www.ombebe.com*
Rosie Hippo: *www.rosiehippo.com*
The Wooden Wagon: *www.thewoodenwagon.com*
Worldwide Child: *www.worldwidechild.com*
Nova Natural Toys & Crafts: *www.novanatural.com*
Giggle: *www.egiggle.com*
Ecobaby Organics: *www.ecobaby.com*
Grembo: *www.grembo.com*
Peppermint: *www.peppermint.com*

beauty

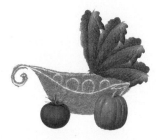

We bet by now you've got a bathroom shelf that contains only nontoxic beauty products, right? If not, turn back to the section on beauty in Part 1 and begin the purge. It's a necessary evil. As you'll probably learn, people tend to give pregnant moms-to-be sweet-smelling belly creams, "soothing" scented candles, and massage oils. Nice gifts, but filled with ingredients you don't want touching you right now. Always read labels and research all new products on the Environmental Working Group's extensive Skin Deep database (*www.ewg.org*) before using. If you're not comfortable throwing products out, less-than-pure items can be given to friends and family, preferably nonpregnant ones.

Some women find pregnancy makes them feel gorgeous. Some don't. Either way, the moment your body stops making sense to you probably isn't the exact moment you'll want to abandon whatever beauty routine you depend on. It's hard enough living without coffee. What follows are some pure and/or organic suggestions to deal with various beauty-related flare-ups you're likely to encounter during your forty weeks.

pimples, bumps, and splotchy skin

In addition to fun changes like bigger boobs and an inflatable belly, pregnancy brings on not-so-desirable rashes and other skin anomalies. Suddenly you're in ninth grade again, and as we discussed in Part 1, Clearasil isn't something you want to be slathering over your face. Tea tree oil doesn't quite pack the same zit-zapping power as its toxic counterparts, but it helps. Try it on its own or in something like Burt's Bees Parsley Blemish Stick (not organic, but very pure). We'd be lying if we didn't admit to stealing our future babies' Weleda diaper cream and dabbing it on a zit now and again. It worked pretty well on ingrown hairs, too. If tea tree oil and diaper cream aren't doing anything for you, it's because the pimples are hormonal by-products, which can be difficult to control when your hormones are running rampant. Keeping your skin clean and exfoliated is always a good idea. Also try using a toner to tighten pores, so they won't let as much dirt in.

stretch marks

Everyone and her mother (and her grandmother) will be warning you about stretch marks from the minute they learn your news. Who knows what helps—some women get red welty versions even when they've slathered them religiously with cream, while some women never see so much as the smallest shiny sliver. If we can do anything to avoid them, we like to. If you can stand oil, use oil. (Some people find it too, well, oily.) Some very organic companies make pregnancy oils (Weleda and Primavera, to name two we've tried). If you prefer a specific scent, try rose, lavender, calendula (which is great for babies, too), or even olive oil. The point is to keep the turkey (your growing belly) basted. Don't forget to grease the sides of your hips, your breasts, and even your butt. Again, we can't promise you that moisture means you won't get marks, but it can't hurt. Some women don't start the oiling until they feel their stomach expanding. Most people report the stretch marks arrive sometime during the second trimester. It can't harm you to start earlier and it might even preempt what could happen during an unexpected growth spurt. If your tummy skin feels tight and itchy, resist the urge to scratch and lube it up instead.

OILS TO AVOID WHEN PREGNANT

Some people say essential oils that mimic a hormonal response should be avoided as a precautionary measure during pregnancy. We haven't seen the hard evidence but are happy to avoid the following just in case. (Herbs used to season food are safe in that capacity.)

- basil
- camphor
- hyssop
- pennyroyal
- sage
- savory
- thuja
- wintergreen
- clary sage
- rosemary
- juniper
- thyme
- bay leaf
- tarragon
- aniseed

candles

In keeping with our smell rule, scented candles aren't good for you either. Even though they rarely have labels to let you be the judge, it's not really a huge surprise. Candles are usually made of paraffin, which is a nonrenewable petrochemical that releases fumes when burned. These fumes have been found to cause kidney and bladder tumors in laboratory animals. Candles also tend to contain a huge amount of artificially fragranced oil that shouldn't be burned and inhaled. Another problem with some candles is that their wicks contain lead. The idea of breathing lead soot is enough to make us forsake ambiance, but luckily we don't have to; there are safe, equally attractive candles out there.

These include beeswax (find ones that aren't bleached or tinted with artificial colors), soy (made from soybean oil), bayberry, and tapioca wax candles. It's easy to find good ones online. Debra Lynn Dadd, the author of *Home Safe Home*, maintains a comprehensive list of candle companies on her Web site: *www.debraslist.com*.

hair dye

If you can go natural for the next nine months, great. If not, know that there is no such thing as organic hair dye. There are, however, safer ways of coloring your hair. At John Masters Salon in New York City (he has a great line of organic hair care available online at *www.johnmasters.com* and at *www.saffronrouge.com*—the curly-haired should really try his lavender and avocado conditioner), Masters does the purest version of dying possible. His dyes are ammonia-free, herbal-based, and have fewer PPDs (para-phenylenediamines—the chemical that creates color and is widely thought to be carcinogenic) than normal ones do. They contain hydrogen peroxide, but they don't contain lead, toluene, or coal tar. Henna is the only option considered more pure, but as Masters points out, it's very limited. It doesn't lighten and doesn't cover gray well. The only natural henna is bright orange red; the others contain metallics. And, believe it or not, not everyone looks good with bright orange hair.

If you must dye, don't do it at home. Masters encourages his clients to wait until after the first trimester. Talk to your hairdresser about the possibility of "organic" highlights or lowlights to tide you over. These procedures don't place the dye in contact with the scalp.

Unfortunately, you'll want to completely avoid dying areas not on your head. Facial bleaching creams, which tons of us use to lighten what we perceive as darkish hair on our upper lips, are a horrible idea, especially when you're pregnant. Masters refuses to put anything on the skin or near the mouth.

Oh, and another thing: perms and hair straightening are also a no-no. But you knew we were going to say that. Too many chemicals.

It's All in Your Head

BY LEXY ZISSU

I wish I knew this when I was a self-conscious teenager, but nobody really looks at you. I'm not saying we're invisible. But no one scrutinizes you the way you scrutinize yourself. Try to remember the color of the shirt your best friend was wearing the last time you saw her. Most likely you can't. When I got pregnant, I jokingly bet a few of my work friends that some of the higher-ups wouldn't even notice I was pregnant until about six months, if even. I don't know if I believed it myself. But sure enough there were plenty of people I saw every day for months and months who didn't quite look closely enough at me to figure it out until there was no way around it. It was a bit shocking, actually. I mean I thought I looked hugely pregnant. But plenty of people didn't even notice.

This lack of attention could have felt bad. I found it useful. It made it easier for me when I had to give up a number of beauty products I felt very attached to, things I was sure I would look horrible without. But if people didn't notice the balloon bursting out of my shirt, then surely a pimple or two, or frizzy hair, or my concern that I reeked as I switched to organic deodorant couldn't possibly be making an impression on them.

I recently e-mailed Deirdre the list of all of the beauty products I have given up since my transitioning phase (which began several years ago when I became more and more interested in organics outside of food). I'm not much of a beauty-product junkie—I don't dye my hair or wear lipstick every day—so I was amazed by how long the list was. Some of the toxic products I had held on to from before I was pregnant were easy to give up once pregnant—they smelled too harsh or too sweet or just made me feel sick. But others were harder to let go of. I'll start at the top (my hair) and work my way down: I gave up several hair conditioners; over-the-counter pimple cream; facial bleach; eye creams with alpha hydroxies and way too many ingredients I couldn't pronounce; face moisturizers also with ingredients I couldn't pronounce, plus preservatives; sunblock; body creams; perfume; prescriptions from my dermatologist; antiperspirant; hydrocortisone cream; nail polish and nail polish remover; cuticle cream; and depilatory cream. I've even changed dental floss. I'm currently pushing for new toothpaste, but my boyfriend has objected to every natural brand so far. I haven't given up anything I didn't find a good organic replacement for, with the exception of the prescription excema cream I was addicted to and which was completely unsafe for pregnant women.

It's hard to use a product if you're convinced something else could be doing the job better, but the pros and cons are a no-brainer. I'm not saying all of my new products are perfect. The sunblock I now use is too greasy. Organic makeup is seriously lacking, especially the foundations, which come in unsubtle skin tones—too yellow, too pink, only one shade of brown (if that). And I missed my pedicures something awful over the summer. The bare nails—even professionally buffed to a shine—were humiliating. They don't fill out a cute sandal the way red toes do. But I got by. And the humiliation was mine alone. I'm quite sure that if my swollen stomach turned no heads, the photo intern—or even my editor—never even noticed my feet.

manis/pedis

Nail polish contains several of the you-want-to-avoid chemicals discussed in Part 1, including phthalates, which make it both flexible and chip resistant. Certain phthalates are banned in Europe, and some big American companies are starting to pull it out of their nail polishes as well, because research has shown it can cause cancer and/or reproductive abnormalities in lab animals. A small study suggested baby boys exposed to high levels of the chemical in utero were more likely to exhibit penile anomalies. The FDA still deems the chemical safe, and critics say the studies are too small. We're happy to err on the side of caution. For women who have to have tidy fingers and toes during their forty weeks, we suggest heading to a well-ventilated salon and asking for a buffing manicure and pedicure. You're trimmed and trussed as usual, but instead of painting your nails with polish, the aesthetician buffs your nails to a high shine. This most likely has its drawbacks, too, but at least none of them are chemical.

phthalates

You're probably getting the picture by now; even though they're everywhere, phthalates should be avoided (see page 36). They're used in everything from fragrance, lotion, shampoo, and hair spray, to insect repellent, detergent, flexible plastic, and food packaging. A 2000 study by the Centers for Disease Control and Prevention found that more than 75 percent of Americans tested had traces of phthalates in their urine. Unfortunately, manufacturers are not required to list the word phthalates on their labels. They can just include them as "fragrance." Meanwhile, pure, organic essential oils are also required to be listed as "fragrance," so the fact is, avoiding phthalates can be tricky. Opt for products you know to be pure whenever possible. And don't hesitate to contact a manufacturer or go to *www.nottoopretty.org* or *www.safecosmetics.org*.

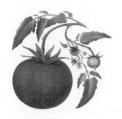

special section—
giving birth

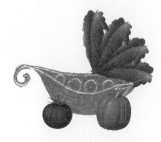

So all of this careful eating and avoiding bleach, paint, and hair dye is for a very good reason: you're having a baby. How you decide to give birth is an extremely personal decision. Whatever choice you make will be a good one. Of course, it's a much more emotional decision than glass versus plastic; it's something you'll want to read about, think about, and plan down to the last detail. There are a bevy of birth books on the market, depending on what route you want to go—hospital, birth center within a hospital (a great option for women who want a more natural experience but aren't comfortable being too far from an operating room), birth center, or home birth. We've weighed in on a few of the less personal decisions you're going to have to make—classes, medical information about drugs, and a last-minute checklist for your delivery.

We live in a country and an era where medicalized birth is standard practice. If you truly want a natural birth, set yourself up for it. Opt for a midwife over an obstetrician, or find an OB who believes in natural childbirth, even for first-time mothers. Then get an education on natural childbirth that includes various non-medicinal pain-coping techniques that go way beyond traditional breathing exercises. If you have to have a hospital birth for a medical reason, or if there are no midwives near you, it's still incredibly important to learn as much as possible about what you're about to go through. Even in a hospital, you can have control over decisions you may have assumed were up to the medical staff in charge.

Books and birth classes can fill you in on exactly how much say you really have in this process. It can be jarring how much this education can feel like preparing for a battle with your health care providers, but these are battles you will never regret. When reading up on a topic—from postdelivery eye ointment to epidurals and the question of whether they can cross your placenta—try to find the actual studies, rather than summaries of them. Too often reporters and writers quoting studies have their own agendas. You may be surprised how different the raw facts are from an article based on the raw facts.

Throughout the learning process, don't feel like you need to rush into a decision, and keep your mind open. Moms and couples often carefully construct birth plans, down to the minutest detail, of how they want their special day to go, but your body and your baby will have their own plans. There is no controlling that, organically or otherwise. If you don't want pain meds but can't stand the pain and have to take them, or if for whatever reason a C-section turns out to be medically necessary, don't beat yourself up. We've interviewed women who say that they felt part of their postpartum depression had to do with the fact that their dream birth plans went awry. They couldn't shake the feeling it was their fault. There is no reason to be disappointed by things beyond your control. Any way she winds up entering the world, the end goal is the same: your baby is with you on the outside. And that's about as organic as it gets.

Birth Class Cliff Notes

BY HALLIE GREIDER

Excellent childbirth classes can certainly exist in various environments—your birth location (hospital or birth center), an independent education center, or in a series taught by a private educator. As a certified childbirth educator and labor support doula, I know how seriously women should and do take childbirth class, and so I would like to offer some recommendations of my own.

To begin with, a series should be taken that ends prior to the onset of the thirty-seventh week of pregnancy. If you can interview your instructor before choosing a class, be sure to ask about their certification process, their motivation for teaching, some of their goals for the class, and what they hope families will walk away knowing that they didn't before. More specifically, talk to them about their underlying message or agenda. How do they feel about using pain medication for labor and birth? What kinds of coping strategies do they practice? How will they prepare you to move into labor? How will partners and additional support people attending the class be incorporated? I also recommend that you ask to speak to a few families that have attended the series. How did they feel this class prepared them? Was it relevant to their experience? Was it helpful?

Typically, an in-hospital childbirth-preparation class is the one most families choose. It's conveniently located in their birth location, and it's usually given by a member of the staff familiar with the hospital, which can be reassuring. Unfortunately, that sense of security is often a false one. Many in-hospital classes lack a focus on individual choices and, most important, evidence-based care (rooted in recent studies). These classes have a tendency to educate families about what to expect upon arrival at the birth location, but not about their options and preferences once they arrive. Moreover, some hospital-based classes reflect the institutions' policies and are more focused on creating compliancy than on helping patients achieve their individual goals.

Out-of-hospital childbirth-preparation classes frequently offer a broader picture of the labor and birth process and the choices that are available to laboring mothers and their partners. Often they are run by educators who include evidence-based information in their classes. They teach families about the risks and benefits of a myriad of choices and empower them to make the best decisions in the individual circumstances of their labors and births. Of course, these kinds of instructors can be found in hospitals as well.

Birthing classes should empower you with knowledge—about the birth process and about yourself. You need to take the time to return to your instincts and inner self and realize that for the most part you already have what you need to bring to this labor and birth. Childbirth classes should help you see your inherent pain-coping abilities and reframe them within a context of labor and birth—"What will I do contraction after contraction?" The classes should also help you crystallize your desires for the birth experience and create a simple birth plan that expresses your preferences. They should ultimately allow you to make the best decisions possible in whatever circumstances that may arise.

For your partner, a good childbirth class can help them see that they know you best, and that they have a valuable role in the birth experience. The classes should give your partner hands-on experience helping you with various positions and coping techniques. They can be a forum for expressing specific fears or concerns about not being the family member in labor, and about how to be as empowering as possible in the support role.

When I was pregnant with my first child during the summer of 2000, I, like many other mothers-to-be, spent endless hours reading books, surfing Web sites, and talking to others. I was well aware that giving birth would be a pivotal experience in my life; I just didn't know to what degree! What it did was help me redefine who I was as a woman and define who I would be as a mother. As a woman, the birth helped me gain a deeper, more profound understanding of what women's bodies are capable of doing. When my newborn son was placed on my chest, I found myself overwhelmed with how much power, strength, and beauty lies within a woman and her body. Undoubtedly, it was that birth experience that motivated me to become involved in the birthing community.

Birthing a child is a natural, normal, instinctive process with which the modern world seems to have lost touch. Today, it is too often seen as something that is done to a woman, rather than by a woman. Childbirth education is essential in debunking that falsehood and critical in helping women and their partners reclaim knowledge and an awareness that was once very common. The goal of a good childbirth class should be to leave you so well informed that you will be able to make decisions confidently—whatever the circumstances.

HALLIE GREIDER works as a childbirth educator and labor support doula in New York City. You can read more about her work on her Web site, www.halliegreider.com.

types of childbirth education classes

Though movies make it seem like the only childbirth education choice is Lamaze, there are many different methods to choose from. These days many women are opting for classes that mix as many of these traditional methods as possible. This gives you the widest range of coping techniques when you go into labor. If you can't find a mix-and-match class, here are the methods usually taught. Always keep in mind that your class is as much about the instructor as it is the method. Hopefully you'll stumble on a great teacher.

LAMAZE

Started in the early 1960s by Dr. Ferdinand Lamaze, this organization was the beginning of the idea that women could do something to help themselves during labor. The method incorporated the actual preparation of women and taught them various coping techniques. Today, Lamaze has evolved into teaching a more comprehensive philosophy—not just patterned breathing techniques. One caveat: sometimes, when taught in very structured hospital settings, Lamaze classes might not provide moms-to-be with enough information. For more, visit *www.lamaze.org.*

BRADLEY

Dr. Robert Bradley introduced the husband/partner into the birthing room. He believed that the partner could and should be involved in the labor and birth. The Bradley classes call the partners "coaches," and there is a heavy (some might say intense) emphasis on birthing without medication. A downside is that women who have studied this method, and for whatever reason go on to have to have a medicated birth or a C-section, often report feeling like they failed at childbirth. Couples interested in Bradley might want to supplement their classes with reading about pain medication just in case. For more information visit *www.bradleybirth.com.*

HYPNOBIRTHING

This philosophy teaches hypnosis techniques to help women reduce fear and tension with the belief that it allows women to have a safer, easier, and more comfortable birth. Many people take these classes as a supplement to a more traditional series to be certain they acquire enough broad information about labor and birth. For more information visit *www.hypnobirthing.com.*

BIRTHING FROM WITHIN

This method was started by Pam England. It is a more soulful, hands-on approach taught through dialogues, birth art, and various group and individual exercises. England has written a book of the same name that encapsulates her philosophy and can obviously be used whether you attend this style of class or not. For more information visit *www.birthingfromwithin.com.*

WATER BIRTHING

Many women say that warm water makes labor pains somewhat easier to handle. Women who have home births usually do so in special tubs, delivering baby from one fluid environment (them) to another (the water). Birthing centers often have whirlpool baths or large tubs (big enough for a partner to get in for support) available, but hospitals tend to have only showers. For information on tub rentals and everything water birthing, check out *www.waterbirth.org.*

Turn the Feet Around

BY ALEXANDRA JACOBS

One morning around twenty-eight weeks into my pregnancy, I became concerned that the baby-to-be wasn't moving enough, and scurried to my OB's group practice in Beverly Hills for an ultrasound. The doctor on call informed me that my amniotic fluid was on the low side, and that the baby was a footling breech: head up, with the feet presenting at the bottom (which explained a strong, intermittent sensation that someone was tap-dancing on my cervix). "With low fluid and breech, I can tell you which way this is going to go," he said. The phrase C-section hovered menacingly in the air. My husband and I looked at each other, aghast.

We'd been planning an all-natural, medication-free birth, attending classes in the Bradley Method, which focuses on good nutrition, deep-breathing techniques, earthy squats, and pelvic rocks. Now it seemed all this diligent preparation might be for naught. Ever since a 2000 study by the Canadian Institutes of Health Research concluded that breech babies delivered by cesarean section were three to four times less likely to die or have serious neonatal problems than those delivered vaginally, few doctors in the United States endorse the latter option—especially not with a footling, the rarest kind, because it is most likely to result in horrors such as "head entrapment " (honey, you don't even want to know) and umbilical cord prolapse, when the cord slips out too early and is vulnerable to dangerous compression. (They are more likely to consider vaginal delivery if the baby is frank breech, or butt-first, because the plumper presenting part allows for easier dilation of the cervix.) I was a footling breech myself, arriving without incident in 1972; my mother would always proudly describe how easily I "walked out," much to the surprise of the attending residents. But I was her second child. Breech births are riskier propositions for first-time mothers, and in the hospital often require large episiotomies and heavy epidurals—the very interventions we'd been hoping to avoid with Bradley.

My regular OB pooh-poohed his colleague's dire prediction. "There's plenty of time for it to turn," he said. About 20 percent of babies are breech at twenty-eight weeks, 15 percent at thirty-two weeks, and only 3 to 4 percent at term. Still, we wanted to do everything possible to maximize these excellent odds. After trawling the Internet and consulting members of the midwife mafia, I began adding a selection of exercises to my daily repertoire. These included lying on the floor with my hips elevated on an ironing board slanted across the bed (an undignified posture known as the "breech tilt"); doing handstands and turning somersaults in the pool of the local Y, to the dismay of the lap-swimmers there; and—most ridiculously of all—having my husband play music, shine a flashlight at, and speak gentle entreaties to the lower part of my womb. All of these made me laugh. None of them worked.

A few weeks later, I found myself sitting in a dimly lit treatment room with orange-painted walls and Norah Jones playing softly in the background, as a gentle-voiced acupuncturist named Tatiana held two burning sticks of mugwort root on either side of my pinky toes. The technique is known as moxibustion, and it stinks to high heaven, but a 1998 study in *The Journal of the American Medical Association* found that it corrected about 25 percent more breech presentations than a control group. In theory, moxibustion is supposed to make the fetus more active and thus interested in flipping, but if anything, mine seemed more sluggish following the treatments; this was unsurprising to me, as the odor of the substance was strikingly reminiscent of collegiate marijuana.

After three unsuccessful sessions, Tatiana suggested we pay a call to a visiting group of indigenous Maori healers who were issuing treatments at a house called the Faerie Wood Ranch in Topanga Canyon. "Hey, when in California . . . ," I thought. The ranch was an idyllic pink medieval-style house with a gorgeous pool and views of the canyons, punctuated by the distant sound of neighing horses, as well as frantic, if perhaps transcendental, moaning from inside the residence. Sprawled on the lawn were people in various stages of blissed-out recovery (or so I assumed) and an assortment of gamboling dogs.

Fifteen minutes later I was lying on a massage table as a tribal elder named Papa Joe, an enormous man with a thick dark beard and bad teeth, pushed and prodded at my belly, assisted by a woman named Anna, who said she was a former nurse at high-risk births. Eventually Papa Joe placed my hand on the baby's head, which I previously had felt somewhere to the right of my navel. It was now underneath my sternum—on its way somewhere, but where? I burst into tears.

Papa Joe backed off fast, perhaps sensing I wasn't a willing candidate for his ministrations. "The baby will go where it wants to go," he said sagely. One hundred fifty dollars lighter but weighted down with guilt, I fled the premises, feeling immense relief as my cervix got kicked (reprovingly?) on the way home.

From what I can judge, the Maoris were trying an unauthorized type of "external cephalic version (ECV)"—basically, when obstetricians attempt to manipulate the fetus into the proper position from the outside. It has about a 60 percent success rate. Because of the small but very frightening risk of premature rupture of membranes, fetal distress, and other complications, it is highly recommended ECV take place in a hospital, when the pregnancy is thirty-seven weeks (term, but the baby is still small enough to have room to move), with facilities for an emergency cesarean at the ready. Amniotic fluid levels should be normal.

Thanks to compulsive water-guzzling, my fluid measurements had gone up significantly, and my OB, after laughing at my trauma in Topanga, cleared the way for an official ECV a few weeks later at Cedars-Sinai Medical Center. After the voodoo vibe of the Maoris, there was something immensely reassuring about checking into the hospital, filling out forms, and being hooked up to a fetal monitor for hours. My doctor drizzled warm mineral oil on my belly and, with the help of a resident, attempted some Papa Joe–esque Rolfing maneuvers—this time, though, the procedure was guided by ultrasound, with heartbeat checks every few moments.

After four attempts, they gave up. My stubborn little baby was simply not budging, and the doctor indicated there might be a structural reason for it—like a short umbilical cord or a malformation of the uterus. The chances of the baby turning on its own at this point, he said, were next to nil.

Josephine arrived via scheduled C-section a little over a week late[...], all the worry she'd caused: pink and screaming, with a perfectly round [...] kling little toes that she likes to kick up while nursing (oh, and the doctors c[...] reason for her "malpresentation"—the first of many mysteries with which my d[...] will presumably present me; I like to think she just had the sense not to dive headfirst [...] this cruel world). It was far from the natural birth I'd wanted, but the baby exceeded my wildest dreams, and in the end, isn't that all that matters?

ALEXANDRA JACOBS is an editor for The New York Observer *and a contributing writer for* Elle *magazine who has also written for* The New York Times, Allure, *and* Harper's Bazaar, *among other publications.*

birth plans

A birth plan is a guide that is written before labor that describes exactly how the event should unfold. There are a million things to consider—sample birth plans can be found online at *www.birthplan.com.* They're more common with midwife types, and with people who use doulas, but hospitals have come to expect them and often ask for a copy upon arrival. Sometimes couples can go overboard—a doctor we know showed us one that was twenty-two pages long. We don't address all of the options here, but they can cover everything from pubic hair shaving to fetal monitoring to drugs, episiotomies, mirrors, photography, cord cutting, and immediate postdelivery care. Our advice is keep the birth plan short—one page of around five basics. These points should include the things that are important to you that are outside the protocol of your hospital or birth location. A good general catchall is: "We want to be informed of all procedures that will happen to Mom and baby." Asking to be informed beforehand (barring any emergency) can help avoid blunders like getting an induction injection of Pitocin (a form of oxytocin) and being told of it as the needle is entering the skin. Unfortunately, this can happen.

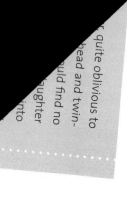

)R THE HOSPITAL/BIRTHING
CENTER TOUR

- ...lure?
- ...es to patients?
- ...sections and epidurals?
- ...nitoring during labor?
- ...or tubs available? Will you be allowed in them
- ...al monitoring?
- ...during labor? Usually you can in a birthing center.
- ...t up to your doctor. Discuss in advance. Labor is
- ...rk.
- What are ... of the room—TV, tape player, rocking chair?
- Can you dim the lights?
- Can you close the door for privacy?
- Can you control the flow of residents in and out of your room (if it is a teaching hospital)?
- Is there a lactation consultant on staff, and will she be on call if necessary?
- What are visiting hours?
- Can partners stay overnight in double rooms? Many hospitals don't allow this, which is beyond our comprehension—how can you break up a family's first night together?
- If not, are private rooms available so your partner can stay with you?
- If so, what do they cost and how much will your health care company cover?
- Can you bring in your own food after delivery?
- How long is the stay expected to be?

doulas

Lots of women choose to hire doulas (a labor coach, basically) to help them through their labor. Not only is a doula with you full-time throughout the entire process (which your OB will most likely not be), but they've been through countless births before. They know of many tricks to help you through the contractions and pain. They'll rub you (even stimulate your nipples!), coach you, and encourage you. They're probably most important in hospital settings, where they can advocate when and if interventions are suggested that may not be medically necessary (yet). We've yet to hear anyone complain about her doula. Most of the women we know who hired them were more than happy to have them there. But we also know plenty of moms who had very supportive labor coaches in their partners and the nurses on labor and delivery. The downside of doulas is that they're pricey. It all depends on where you live, but they can cost well over a thousand bucks (this usually includes help drafting a birth plan, labor, and a postpartum home visit). If it isn't an expense you can afford, we're sure you'll do just fine without one. But if you have some extra cash, they can be amazing. Think of the money that could be saved in the long run by insurance companies if they covered doulas as an alternative to epidurals. To find a doula near you, check out *www.dona.org* (Doulas of North America).

packing for labor

Every pregnancy Web site, friend, and mother-in-law has a list of what is essential for your stay at the hospital. This includes what you need to wear and have, and what the baby needs to wear and have to go home (a car seat, for example). Wade through the advice and pick and choose what makes sense to you. It does seem that what a baby needs most is a swaddling blanket and a breast. Here are a few ideas we thought might be helpful:

- A birthing ball (great for finding "comfortable" positions while in labor). Just air it out in advance if it is new; you don't want to be smelling PVC as you labor.
- A yoga mat.
- Tennis balls—good for counterpressure and massage.
- Snacks—nothing too heavy (some women get very nauseated in active labor), but high-energy organic goodies like nuts, dried fruit, and carrots are good. If your room has a freezer, you could also bring ice pops. Many birth coaches will suggest power bars. It's not exactly food, but

then again some women say lollipops have helped them through. If a little high-fructose corn syrup helps you now, go for it. Don't forget snacks for your partner. This could take a while, and they need to keep their energy up, too.

- A copy of your birth plan, insurance card, and any hospital paperwork you've already filled out.
- Your marriage certificate if you and your partner don't have the same last name (according to individual state law).
- Water and other drinks. You need to keep hydrated and you might not like their choice of water, or be given water when you need it.
- Music—if it soothes you.
- If you're modest, an old skirt or slip that has slits up the sides (so you don't have to reveal more than you want to in a backless hospital gown).
- Socks.
- Layers. You'll be hot and cold.
- Something to keep your hair back.
- Lip balm—all that breathing can chap your lips.
- Camera with film or an extra memory card, and batteries.
- A bathing suit and flip-flops for your partner if they want to get in the shower or bath with you.
- Cell phone chargers (if cell phones are allowed).
- Money—including small bills and change for vending machines.

bringing on labor

If your due date comes and goes, your doctor may start talking to you about induction. Some providers will allow you to get to forty-two weeks before suggesting this, but the universal cutoff point is getting closer to forty-one weeks. There are two medications commonly used to ripen your cervix: Cytotec and Cervidil. Cervidil is basically a string coated in prostaglandin, which is laced around your cervix for twelve hours. Cytotec is actually an ulcer medication and is not FDA-approved for cervix softening, but it is widely used for this purpose anyway. It comes in pill form, which you can take orally or insert vaginally. Here are some nonmedical ideas that are also thought to encourage labor.

If you try them, be sure to run it by your health care provider—especially the herbs and oils.

- Sex: orgasm releases oxytocin, which stimulates contractions. Semen is high in prostaglandin, the very same thing in Cervidil.
- Evening primrose oil: 500 mg two to three times daily.
- Red raspberry leaf tea.
- Massage and acupuncture. There are certain spots on the body that are thought to encourage labor if stimulated. We know a few women who said their labor was brought on by prompting of the ankle.
- Castor oil stimulates the bowel and possibly the uterus. (It will most certainly give you diarrhea and may or may not bring on labor—so think twice.)
- There are several herbs thought to bring on labor. This needs to be discussed with an herbalist, and not without the input of your OB or midwife. For solid herb information check out Susun Weed's Web site, *www.susunweed.com*, or her book *Wise Woman Herbal for the Childbearing Year*.
- A doctor or a midwife can strip your membranes, which is a technique used to induce labor by placing a finger within the cervix and running it around the inside to separate the membranes from the lower uterine area.

If your cervix is already softened, or these things help it to soften, doctors may also want to intervene to kick-start contractions. Most often this is done with Pitocin, which is basically synthetic oxytocin. If you're not ready to go this route (some people worry Pitocin can slow down labor, not speed it up, and create a snowballing need for other drugs), ask your doctor if you can try nonmedicinal stimulation first. Generally this includes either stimulating the nipples (which is thought to release your own oxytocin), walking around, or rocking in a rocking chair to try to get the baby's head to hit your cervix.

When to Say When

BY BETH WISHNIE

After being a labor doula, birth educator, and massage therapist who specializes in prenatal and perinatal massage for ten years, I was finally ready to embark on motherhood. I had "experienced" so many labors, providing comfort and support to moms-to-be, that I felt that nothing could surprise me during my own labor. In my mind, I could piece together bits of other comfort measures that worked best in other women's labors to create what would be my perfect birth. I knew how to labor at home as long as possible to get to the hospital almost ready to push. I knew how I wanted the hospital room to look to create the coziest environment, what kinds of music felt right, what positions worked best during labor and pushing, what kind of food I would eat to keep my blood sugar and energy level up.

Even reading this now, I am laughing at the insanity of my thought process. I have never seen a birth go exactly as planned. In every birth class and before each birth, I emphasize the importance of becoming educated enough to make choices about what's important to you, but not to be wedded to a plan, because until you're in labor, you don't know how you're going to feel or how the baby will ultimately choose to come into the world. I somehow believed I was more in control than any of the eighty or ninety mothers I had seen in labor because—well—I guess I just got cocky because I thought I knew so much.

So I was a little surprised at thirty-eight weeks that my labor seemed to be starting. I was woken up by a big contraction and lost my plug early in the morning. By the time I got to the doctor's appointment I had later that morning, my water broke.

Well, at least I could be in control of how the rest of the day would go. I planned to go home and experience early labor in my favorite environment. But my doctor's office was actually in the hospital where I was going to deliver and the doctor felt I should be a "direct admit." I didn't agree. I explained that this wasn't how my labor was supposed to go. I had been with plenty of women whose water broke and we stayed at home and took their temperature for hours to watch for infection before they were ready to go to the hospital. But somehow, I was on my way to the labor and delivery room without any real contractions.

At least I got to make my room look the way I wanted it to. I had plenty of time to sit around and wait for my contractions to get noticeable. My nurse was joking with me about how low-maintenance I was because my birth plan stated I wanted no intervention of any kind. She was very low-key and ready to leave me alone for the day after she took my temperature and blood pressure for her charts.

Well, I was in for my next surprise. My blood pressure was unbelievably high. Usually my pressure is around 110/70 and today it was at 180/90. My cool and calm nurse started to talk in clipped sentences and stuck me in a bed on my back with monitors wrapped all around me. I explained to her that this wasn't how my labor was supposed to go. She didn't care what I thought. She saw preeclampsia starting and was doing her job. I tried to lie on my side to get my blood pressure down, and my now panicky nurse yelled at me to stop self-treating and get back on my back.

Of course, while I was on my back, my contractions started to kick in. Not the greatest position to be in. My doctor was paged, and I pleaded with her to help me. Luckily, none of the other hard-core signs of preeclampsia were setting in. I didn't have a headache and there was no protein in my urine. The doctor said if I could get one good blood pressure reading, I could get off my back and out of bed. My husband and I closed our eyes and thought positive thoughts about low numbers each time the blood pressure cuff tightened around my arm. Finally, somehow, I got a 135/80 and I was freed.

I decided I'd get back to my plan. My contractions were incredibly intense now and hurt more than I ever thought they would. I put on my tape of ocean sounds and focused on relaxing my body during contractions. But they got closer and closer together and lasted longer and longer until the contractions were lasting six minutes and I was only getting twenty-second breaks. And I was having back labor. This wasn't how my labor was supposed to go.

So now the calm, experienced doula, birth educator, and massage therapist was screaming loud enough for the patrons at Jerry's Deli across the street to hear. And I was digging my nails into my husband's arm, hyperventilating, and dreading the contractions as they pounded me.

After sixteen hours of the incessant rolling, piercing pain, I decided to throw my birth plan out the window and ask for an epidural at seven to eight centimeters. My husband tried to question me because he knew how strongly I felt about getting through labor without any intervention. And as far as he knew, I was supposed to be in control. I gave him a look that he understood quickly and within minutes the anesthesiologist was next to me. I told him I wanted a walking epidural in one of my twenty-second breaks, and he said he didn't think that would be enough. But this felt like the one thing I had to hold on to. I wanted to feel enough to understand what a body goes through in the last stage of labor so I could help my clients in a whole new way.

For an hour and a half, I got a kind of break. I could still feel pain, but the torpedo coming out of my rear end pulled back just a little. At least I didn't have to scream. When the medicine ran out, it was about time to push. I had pictured myself squatting while I pushed, but I was too worn out to move out of my bed. Instead, I stayed on my side and held a leg in the air. This wasn't how my labor was supposed to go. But fifty minutes later, a beautiful little girl was in my arms. And it didn't matter how it was supposed to go.

BETH WISHNIE is a licensed massage therapist specializing in pre- and perinatal massage. She is also a certified birth doula and birth educator.

episiotomy

When it comes to tearing during childbirth, some women naturally do, and some women luckily don't. Still others are given episiotomies, surgical incisions in the perineum (the area of skin between the vagina and anus) to make more room for a baby. Episiotomies are largely performed in hospitals. Birth centers and midwives tend to avoid cutting, relying instead on warm compresses, controlled pushing, perineal massage, and support during delivery. The routine use of episiotomy is a controversial topic within the medical community right now, which makes it hard to figure out for yourself when it's really necessary. This is a discussion you'll want to have prior to birth with your health care provider. Ask them how often they perform episiotomy. If their rate is high, chances are you'll be getting one. Often an OB will say they perform them only "when necessary," so ask them to define necessary. It may be that an OB only performs an episiotomy when a mom looks like she's about to tear badly. Doctors tend to believe episiotomy cuts heal better than severe tears and may even help protect against future incontinence. Midwives disagree and say natural tears heal better, and that episiotomies lead to increased postpartum discomfort and a longer healing time. Though episiotomy can be avoided, as with every other aspect of birth, keep an open mind. There could be a medical emergency (fetal distress, for example) when a surgical snip could be just what you need.

A Tale of Two Births

BY SALLY SCHULTHEISS

My children are two years apart. I did not have pain medication for either birth and, mercifully, neither required any emergency procedures. But the first took place in a birthing center in New York City, the second at a hospital in Los Angeles. What brought the differences between the two experiences into sharp relief were not the dramatic stories that typically define each setting—I wasn't doused in herbs at the birthing center or slapped onto an operating table against my will at the hospital. The first birth didn't happen in a whirlpool, surrounded by friends in dreadlocks who brought their children to watch the "beautiful dance." The second time, no nurse hung over me, epidural drip in hand, saying, "C'mon, you know you want it." So my advice to someone debating between a birthing center and a hospital is not based on safety or health. My question would be: How involved do you want to be in the birth? Are you someone who says, "Give me drugs, the sooner the better"? When you're sick, do you ask your doctor about the antibiotic before you ask about the illness? Or are you someone who thinks that if they don't feel the birth, in all its natural awkwardness and pain, it might as well have not happened at all?

I consider myself to be sort of a preppy hippie. I eat organic but can't be bothered to join the health food co-op down the street. I shave under my arms but don't wear antiperspirant. I wanted a natural birth, but I didn't want to do it at home, and I didn't want an audience. So while there were parts about going to a birthing center, with all its alterna-ness, that didn't feel exactly me, I wanted to get medical attention from people who believe that having a baby without drugs is normal and healthy—not a dangerous experience that could turn deadly at any moment.

I was seeing a fancy uptown gynecologist when I became pregnant with my first child. At eight weeks along, I called her office to set up an appointment and the nurse told me the doctor's policy was not to see any patients until the end of the first trimester. So when the ninety-second day arrived, my husband took the morning off work (not easy for a high school math teacher) and we rode four subways to the doctor's office for an ultrasound. We joked that other than a First Response test in my seventh week, we'd had no real confirmation there was indeed a bun in the oven. Gregg and I held hands as we watched the little lima bean float around inside me, mainly thrilled that twelve weeks of nausea and tight waistbands meant something more than indigestion. Then we met with the doctor—a friendly fortyish redhead who'd recently been quoted in a glossy women's magazine about her successful fertility treatments. She asked us a few questions and then sprinted through a litany of dos and don'ts regarding my diet, exercise, and general habits. She then handed us a stack of pamphlets on a variety of subjects, ranging from the importance of the alpha-fetoprotein test to the "Stork Club," in which members pay an additional fee to get a private room after their delivery. It was a special day, in the way that the beginning of all first pregnancies are. But two weeks later, after researching my options online and deciding that natural was the way I wanted to go, I faxed over a letter to my doctor requesting that all of my records be transferred to the Elizabeth Seton Childbearing Center on West Fourteenth Street.

When we first told people where I was giving birth, the reactions varied. Mothers of one child or more shook their heads in a just-you-wait-and-see-how-much-pain-you're-going-to-be-in way. Single friends seemed to think you were cool for trying but ultimately didn't really care. And for the most part, our families responded with support thinly disguising one unanimous thought: "You're going to die. Smelly hippies are going to kill you and your baby."

I don't really blame them. I mean, we've all heard the horror stories about cords wrapped around necks, failed heartbeats, meconium swallowings, and emergency C-sections. The general consensus these days is that it's good to have lots of doctors and medical equipment around just in case something happens. And even though St. Vincent's Hospital, where I would be taken in case of such an emergency, was just a block and a half away, the mere notion of a birthing center seemed anachronistic to them, almost perverse. Why would you ever choose to give birth in a state of limited medical provisions when today's world had so many to offer? For Gregg's father, who had polio as a child, it was like watching the recent trend to willingly forsake the vaccine. Why take risks you don't have to?

Well, the answer wasn't simply that I don't trust modern medicine. I do, if I'm sick. But to me, pregnancy isn't an illness and doesn't need a whole lot of medical attention. It just happens, and the more you stay out of its way, the better the outcome. The more reading I did, the more I began to believe that a lot of those "emergency" C-sections and other interventions had more to do with the threat of litigation and insurance premiums than with real necessity. I also heard stories about deliveries scheduled around doctor's ski trips, and C-sections bumped up to prevent putting on those last few pounds during the thirty-ninth and fortieth weeks. To me, those stories were uglier.

When Gregg and I went to our first appointment at Elizabeth Seton, he was still a little skeptical of what a birthing center might entail. He knew more would fall on his shoulders as my birth partner, but he wanted to be supportive of my wishes. We were both a little cranky that day; I was late to arrive and Gregg had rushed over on his lunch break, so we slogged through the questionnaire as though we were filling out paperwork at H&R Block. In addition to the expected inquiries about our family medical histories, there were pages and pages of questions about our emotional and mental states. They wanted to know how long we'd been together as well as married, if either of us had a history of depression, and our attitudes on parenting. Then we couldn't help but break out of our bad moods when the nurse asked us to lean toward each other so she could take a Polaroid of us—which went right into our file. The nurse showed me how to weigh myself and enter it on my chart each time I came in for a checkup, and also how to read the "dip," a marker that measures protein, glucose, and water levels in your urine. Each month I would do these routine procedures myself and fill in my chart before seeing the midwife.

When I first went to the hospital after learning I was pregnant with my second child, I went alone and left my husband at home with our fifteen-month-old son, Eddie. (The center closed down four days after I delivered, because it was unable to pay an increase in insurance premiums, and I had moved to Los Angeles.) A stooped-over, older woman led me into a windowless room with several desks lining the walls and asked me a battery of questions about my health, including the last time I ingested alcohol. She weighed me, took my blood pressure, told me I needed to completely quit caffeine (even decaf coffee and tea, which contains trace amounts, she said), and set me up for my next checkup, in a month. My checkups there, over the next several months, would be much different from those at Elizabeth Seton. A nurse performed my dips and weighed me and never told me the results unless I asked.

At the birthing center, over the course of prenatal care, we met with nearly every midwife on staff, each of whom had seemingly endless amounts of time to spend with us, fielding every question, sometimes even just chatting. One midwife met Gregg's usual "Everything okay? Anything to be worried about?" paranoia with a chuckle and said, "You think you're worried now? Wait until they're thirteen and don't call you and you wait up until two A.M., when they stumble in the door." It put everything in perspective and calmed our nerves, if only for a moment. As part of its program, Elizabeth Seton also required that all women have a birth partner and that each couple take a six-week birthing class and two four-hour workshops, one each on newborn care and breastfeeding.

My labor, from the first itty-bitty contraction felt on Tuesday night to the birth of my son at 5:30 A.M. Thursday morning, lasted twenty-eight hours. In that time, my friend Lizzy massaged my lower back with a warm sock full of uncooked rice, my husband, Gregg, talked me through every crest of every labor pain, I lapped Prospect Park on foot, fell asleep for forty-five minutes during acupuncture, took three showers, two soaks in the birthing center whirlpool, drank three liters of water and five packets of Emergen-C, ate half a peanut butter sandwich and two energy bars, traveled between two boroughs, the phone rang fifteen times, and three neighbors asked me, "Are you in labor right now?!" Over the course of my labor, two editions of *The New York Times* were printed and most Manhattanites completed nearly two nights of sleep, attended a full day of work, and ate three meals, plus snacks.

It was an exhausting and excruciating experience, but it was an experience, not a procedure. I wouldn't have done it any other way, but I can't imagine it any other way. And when it was all done, when I was lying there next to my new baby, I felt really macho for not having used any pain meds at all.

My second birth was a blur. And although I know there was a tremendous amount of pain involved, I can barely remember any. I attribute this mostly to it being the second child, to being more than a pound lighter with a smaller head. But I'm almost willing to say that if you're having your second child and have any desire to do it naturally, don't even bother with drugs. When I arrived at the hospital after about five hours of contractions—some strong, some mild—I was eight centimeters dilated. When I'd arrived at the birthing center at the same point with my first child, I was five centimeters. I felt like a fraud! I was sure they were going to send me and my tiny cervix home for another day. But at the hospital, I was so far along that I may not have had time for drugs. "What did you do for pain with your first child?" they asked. "Nothing," I said, and not another word was mentioned. I went straight into the delivery room and two hours later, when contractions were a deceiving fifteen minutes apart, after two pushes, my second child was born.

So what's the moral of the story? Weigh your fears. Are you more afraid of doctors or of pain? Are you interested in experiencing the birth process, or are you interested in getting it over with? I have never heard of a woman who has regretted giving birth in a birthing center. I don't regret giving birth in a hospital either, but I also don't really appreciate it. The midwife and nurse I spent twelve hours with at the birthing center, moving from pool to shower to bed to chair, are integral parts of my memories—I can call up their personalities very clearly. The people who delivered me at the hospital are just a parade of names and faces. So maybe the real question is, how do you want to shape your memories?

SALLY SCHULTHEISS *is a freelance writer living in Los Angeles. She's a contributing writer for* Real Simple *and writes frequently for* Cookie *magazine.*

pain relief

As we said before, birthing classes can teach you a zillion pain-coping techniques, from breathing to positions to massage. We highly recommend you look into classes and learn as much as possible before your big day. Most people in this country opt for drugs to relieve their pain. This can include narcotics and/or an epidural. An epidural is a local anesthetic inserted via catheter into a sac in your spine that numbs you from about your rib cage to your knees. If it works, it can greatly diminish the pain of your contractions.

We can't make this to-drug-or-not-to-drug decision for you. We can only suggest you read as much as possible about it before your water breaks. And, again, keep your mind open. Every woman labors differently. You may think you'll have no problem with natural childbirth, but won't be able to take the pain. Or you may have one of those superfast births that don't even give you enough time to think about pain meds (don't we all wish!). Talk to your OB or midwife about their take on pain medications. Find out what is in the particular epidural cocktail your hospital will be using. This is an area of childbirth where both the medical and midwifery communities' bias is at its strongest (and sometimes ugliest). We encourage you to listen carefully and then make up your own mind.

You've been keeping your baby pretty pure for these nine months, so in some sense it might feel strange to suddenly take drugs while she is still in utero. We think it seems highly unlikely that some amount of whatever drug you take won't cross the placenta and wind up in your baby. When researching epidurals and narcotics, you will likely run across many anecdotal stories of drugs leading to slower labor, bad tearing, and episiotomies for women who can't feel enough to push on their own. And more stories about "sleepy" babies who are less likely to nurse immediately because of the possibility that there are drugs in their teeny systems. You'll also hear about women, exhausted by hours of labor, who can actually nap and recuperate when they have an epidural, leaving them (somewhat) refreshed for the actual delivery and ensuing mayhem. Some women try to control exactly when the drug enters their system—holding off until they are halfway dilated. There has been recent speculation and debate that an epidural administered before this point actually increases the risk of having a C-section. These women try to taper the epidural off at about nine centimeters so they will be able to feel enough to push. Do keep in mind that once you've had an epidural, you won't be walking around. You might have had enough that you can't even move, or if you can, your balance will be faulty and the risk of falling is too great (and not one the hospital will let you take). Also, an epidural always comes with increased monitoring, which many women interested in natural childbirth find too constricting.

In the end, this pain-management decision is yours. Keep your choice private if it makes you more comfortable, or if you feel like you'll be judged if you take drugs. It's not an easy choice. Just remember no matter what you do, the end result will be what you've been waiting for.

Further Reading

- Henci Goer's *Thinking Woman's Guide to a Better Birth* (*www.hencigoer.com*)
- Childbirth Connection (*www.child birthconnection.org*)
- The American College of Obstetricians and Gynecologists (*www .acog.org*)
- Penny Simpkin's *Birth Partner*
- Peggy O'Mara's *Mothering Magazine's Having a Baby, Naturally: The Mothering Magazine Guide to Pregnancy and Childbirth*
- Ina May Gaskin's *Ina May's Guide to Childbirth*
- Pam England's *Birthing from Within: An Extra-Ordinary Guide to Childbirth Preparation*
- Sheila Kitzinger's *Politics of Birth* (*www.sheilakitzinger.com*)

To Each Her Own

BY DR. SIOBHAN M. DOLAN

I never thought that being pregnant was easy. I know some women love being pregnant, but I was never one of them. I love having kids but getting them was hard work.

I was an OB-GYN resident when I had my first two children and an attending obstetrician when I had my third. I can remember throwing up on my way to work at five in the morning, having an amniocentesis with three beepers on the waist of my scrubs, not fitting into my shoes but not having time to go to the store for new ones and wearing my sneakers with the laces open, and I can remember being told not to slouch at the operating room table when I was about thirty-eight weeks pregnant. So I had to work hard for my kids, but the thing I liked about being pregnant was lying in a dark call room and feeling like I had my kids with me. In a funny way, I appreciated my kids' company during my long lonely call nights, long before I had even met them.

Each of my experiences with labor and delivery was unique. With my first, I had an induction at forty weeks because my fluid was low. It was a long induction, over thirty hours, and I had an epidural the moment I started feeling contractions at all. As a result, I didn't feel much of the labor, and my husband and I could focus on the amazing experience of watching our daughter's birth. I had attended many hundreds of births by then, but there is nothing quite like the first time you lay eyes on your own child and hold her in your arms.

With my second, I was also induced for low fluid (occupational hazard of being on my feet all day) and also had an early epidural. But the labor went very quickly and easily. Our second daughter arrived about ten minutes after I got out of a rocking chair because I felt pressure, and she almost beat me to the punch, as she continues to do each day.

After my second daughter was born, I can remember talking to a patient one day. The woman was quite compelling and told me that she was highly committed to giving birth naturally, with no medication or pain relief at all. She told me passionately that giving birth to her children was the most empowering experience of her life and it was what made her really feel like a woman. I felt perturbed by the fact that I didn't feel that way about birthing my own children, and thus with my third child, a son, I decided to go naturally.

Well, life doesn't always go the way you plan. Unfortunately, my son was noted to have an adrenal mass on ultrasound about two weeks before his birth, and thus my best-laid plans for natural delivery were thwarted by my need to know, at forty weeks, if this child would need major surgery to remove one kidney and an adrenal gland within a few weeks of his birth. That thought was unimaginable, but I entered my third induction with the firm mind-set that my son needed to be born, we needed to know the reality of his medical condition, and we needed to proceed with whatever treatment would be necessary.

I was induced, labored naturally, and delivered within twelve hours, with no pain medicine at all. I watched *ER* and *Letterman* and the pain worsened. It was mind over matter for me—the need to know was so strong that I knew I could get through anything. The pains came, but they went, and although I felt empowered by my experience, the physical aspect of the labor and delivery did not turn out to be the most amazing experience of my life. I think some people are more physical than others, and I would say that the greatest accomplishments of my life are based more in the intellectual and emotional world. But I'm glad I experienced natural labor and delivery because now I'll never wonder. And it turned out that the adrenal mass was benign and our son has been completely healthy.

My advice to myself and to patients is to keep an open mind. You can plan your vacation and expect to have it come out pretty much the way you hope, but you cannot plan your labor and delivery and be certain that your plans will come true. Sometimes interventions are needed or medical complications arise, so keeping an open mind can be very useful. Have an epidural if you want, or go naturally if that works for you. Change your mind in the middle of labor or wait and see how you're doing and make your decisions as you go. At the end of the day, there will be many challenges and rewards to having a family, and giving birth is only the beginning. What you really want is to have a healthy mother and a healthy baby, and if you get that, your birthing experience is truly a success.

Dr. Siobhan M. Dolan is an assistant professor of obstetrics and gynecology and women's health at the Albert Einstein College of Medicine/Montefiore Medical Center in New York City.

PART THREE *living*

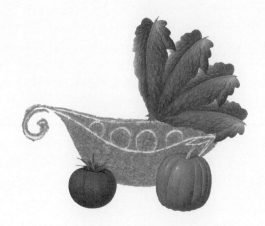

INTRODUCTION

Just because you've had your baby doesn't mean it's time to abandon your organic lifestyle. It's critical that while you're breastfeeding, your diet and everything else you do, wear, and breathe should certainly remain as organic as it has been for the past nine months, which is why we discuss breastfeeding in almost every section of Part 3. What you expose yourself to goes into your baby's milk. And you clearly don't want to revert to using harsh chemicals to clean your home, do your laundry, or weed your garden now that there are newborn nostrils breathing nearby. Having an organic pregnancy results in an organic baby, which means that everything that surrounds her—from crib sheets to diaper cream to the bottles she drinks from—should be organic. When sleep-deprived and getting used to a new way of life, pesticides and toxins may be the last thing you have time to think about. Which is why it's great that living organically is by now second nature or at least close to it. Don't beat yourself up if you run out of chlorine-free diapers and have to use a conventional one from time to time, or if you're starving and stuff whatever packaged thing you can find into your mouth, or if you can't find a day care provider willing to wear your baby in an organic cotton sling. Do what you can. It will be good groundwork for a complete organic childhood.

CHAPTER THIRTEEN

food

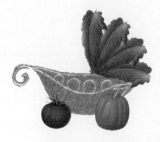

In the hours it takes you to deliver your baby, you naturally morph from host environment to milk truck—unless you're not breastfeeding, in which case see our discussion of organic formula (page 193). Breast milk is the best food for your baby—perfectly suited to nourish infants and protect them from disease. Your diet for both important jobs should remain largely the same. You want your breast milk to be as pure as can be. To produce the healthiest milk, you should continue eating your organic, well-balanced, whole foods diet, filled with fruits and veggies, whole wheats and grains, and plenty of iron- and calcium-rich foods, plus lean proteins. Eat a variety of things so you're sure to hit all of the nutrients you and your baby need, and so you expose your infant to many flavors. Some people think you need to consume more calories to breastfeed than you did when you were pregnant. If you are a person who counts calories, you ate 300 more calories a day when you found out you were pregnant. When breastfeeding, the going thought is that you'll want to add 200 more, for a total of 500. You know how we feel about rigid diets. The fact is, some women get hungrier when breastfeeding; some don't. Just listen to your body.

no-hands eating

There comes a time during your babymoon when you're home alone for the first time. It's scary and exhilarating. It's exhausting and hilarious. And then . . . you're hungry. But you can't put the baby down. If you do, she cries. So you're carrying her around dancing and singing and doing everything you can. But you're really hungry. This is when packaged food starts to look really, really good. Don't give in. A little planning ahead can mean avoiding cookies for lunch. When shopping, buy things you can grab and eat with one hand like bananas, organic raisins, carrots, and nuts (any but peanuts). Or prep food the night before so you won't be stranded. Leave snacks that don't need to be refrigerated near all of the spots where you breastfeed.

breastfeeding

Many women say that breastfeeding is one of the hardest things they've ever done. Set up some support beforehand. Get in touch with people who will encourage you not to give up—lactation consultants, friends, family, La Leche, doulas, other women who have breastfed, your pediatrician, and even your doctor. There are plenty of books written on the subject (for some of our favorites and other great breastfeeding resources, flip to Chapter 15, "Wellness"). We want to encourage you to stick it out. Even if it is hard at first. It is enormously beneficial to your baby. Patience.

what not to eat when breastfeeding

If you were thinking you could hop right back on the smoking, drinking, caffeinated bandwagon the minute you pushed your new bundle out, we're here to dampen your dream. Traces of what you eat and drink do pass into your breast milk. This trio—which are, if you want to get technical about it, drugs not food—should still be avoided. We're not saying a drink from time to time when you're breastfeeding is the end of the world, especially when metabolized with food. If this is something you're interested in doing, you probably want to have only a few drinks per week even with a meal. We have plenty of friends who time their drinking and breastfeeding, or who have mastered the after-party pump-and-dump maneuver. And other friends who cringe at the thought of throwing out liquid gold. We also know women who have started back on tea and/or coffee after birth. Smoking is never permissible, but in terms of caffeine and alcohol, it's all about if it works for the baby. One mom we know couldn't figure out why her kid was crying so much. The culprit was the mother's (unfortunate) addiction to Diet Coke, which she returned to postpartum. She was more than happy to give it up again when she realized nixing the caffeine would help her baby—and ultimately her—sleep better. Check with your lactation consultant, favorite breastfeeding book, or pediatrician for more specific details.

If you have a family history of allergies, peanuts should be avoided while breastfeeding, in order to reduce the risk of your baby developing a peanut allergy—and other allergies—later in life. With food allergies on the rise, most moms, often at their doctor's suggestion, avoid peanuts in the home for a good long while after birth. Some people avoid for one year, others for up to three years. If you haven't already tried other nut butters (like almond and cashew), we suggest you do. They're better than you think.

Other than that, you don't need to avoid anything. Which is pretty liberating considering the restrictions that have been weighing on you for the past nine months. When you were pregnant, what you ate went pretty directly to the baby. Now you're basically filtering your intake before it gets to your kid. It isn't believed that *Listeria*, for example, can pass through breast milk. There was an unheated prosciutto (nitrate-free) and fresh mozzarella sandwich waiting for at least one of us postdelivery. Delish.

Lactose Intolerance: Testing
My Breast Milk

BY FLORENCE WILLIAMS

When my second baby was seven months old, I sent my breast milk halfway around the world to get it tested for pollutants. The Europeans are better than we in this, as in so many things. The Swedes are basically connoisseurs of breast milk. They were the ones who discovered PCBs (a toxic industrial lubricant) in human milk in the 1960s. Always a little late on the safety trends, the United States banned the chemicals a decade later.

Now the Swedes are hot on the trail again. The culprits this time are PBDEs, or polychlorinated biphenyls, a class of fat-loving flame retardants showing up everywhere from seal flesh to lake sediments. When I learned of a breast-milk study out of Texas, I signed up, sending the delicate little vials overnight to a special lab in Germany from my home in Montana. As an environmental journalist, I'd been reading about toxins that accumulate in human tissue, and I was curious to know my own "body burden." I also thought it would be a great way to tell the story of these pollutants in *The New York Times Magazine*, which published it in January 2005.

It took a couple of months to get my results from the fancy spectrographic doohickey machine, and during that time, I pretty much freaked out. I was researching the article, and the more I learned, the worse it all seemed. The world was irredeemably, irrevocably contaminated, we were all exposed, and there wasn't a dang thing we could do about it. I've always fancied myself healthy. I've lived in the Rocky Mountains for most of my adult life, far from smog and concrete. I exercise a lot. I filter my water. I rarely eat red meat, and when I do, it's organic. Since my first pregnancy, four years ago, I've bought ridiculously expensive organic produce, hormone-free milk, and natural face creams.

But flame retardants, as with so many persistent organic pollutants, are like the flu: exposure is everywhere, and hiding behind a healthy diet won't guarantee your safety. They are also a leveler of socioeconomic class. Californians, in many ways the healthiest Americans, appear to harbor the highest body burden of flame retardants. This is because the state has the highest fire safety standards and people's homes are oozing with the stuff. But California has affected—or infected—us all as state standards become the norm for manufacturers nationwide. On average, Americans have 100 times greater the amount of PBDEs in their systems as people elsewhere in the world.

So I knew I would be carrying some. PBDEs are not bonded molecularly to their products. They are likely sitting on your computer casings and television sets, in your carpets and carpet padding, in your household dust bunnies and in your laundry lint filter, on your windows, on your roofing tiles, in your mattress pads and your furniture upholstery, in your food, your milk, and maybe even in your vegan smoothies. Eco-goddesses, beware.

Hence my freak-out, just as, dear reader, you may be freaking out now. I began eyeing my house suspiciously. My beloved comfortable couch, refuge of my third trimester? Got 'em. My flat-screen computer monitor? Yep. And what about the other nasty chemicals I was also reading about? Phthalates in my kids' toys? Yep. Parabens in my sunscreen? Check. Perchlorate, a jet fuel, on my organic lettuce? Yessirree.

I noticed a strong odor emanating from my son's new beanbag chair, marketed as a "green" product because it was filled with recycled foam polystyrene, otherwise known as Styrofoam. I called the store where we bought it. They had no idea what the odor could be. I called the U.S. Environmental Protection Agency, where a researcher told me he couldn't be sure, but, yes, polystyrene gas emits a strong odor, and, yes, it's toxic. I called a major manufacturer of beanbag chairs. The president of the company told me he would never let his own child sit on a chair made with recycled Styrofoam. The material could have once been used in an industrial process, he said, and furthermore, with the recycled foam all shredded, the polystyrene gas is more volatile and less contained than in the newer, beaded foam. (Tip: Don't buy recycled foam. Or, better, do what I eventually did, despite feeling a bit ridiculous, and replace the polystyrene with organic buckwheat hulls.)

This all made me furious. As mothers, as consumers, as pregnant women trying our hardest to nurture a little being with ten toes and a high IQ and a decent shot in a complicated world, we were inadvertently siphoning them neurotoxins, carcinogens, and who knows what else (and, believe me, we know very little). None of these products or foodstuffs came with warning labels or ingredients lists. No beanbag said, "Yo, by the way, better not let your toddler sit on this."

Increasingly, our world is so toxic that we require additional toxics to protect us from the existing toxics. We need flame retardants to protect us from all the highly flammable plastics in our homes. Consider environmentally triggered diseases like asthma that require pharmaceuticals to ameliorate. The pharmaceutical by-products, in turn, end up in our water supply and in the tissues of invertebrates and fish. Pesticides and antibiotics require ever stronger and new formulations to stay one step ahead of evolving bugs. Both inadvertently hit expanding targets. The notion of "toxic trespass" is not one the founding fathers envisioned. One farmer's chicken's drug could end up making her neighbor's strep infection untreatable. A factory emission from Milwaukee ends up in someone's liver in Weehawken.

It's a cycle I never thought much about until it became clear my breasts were part of it.

Not only do we have no way of knowing what we consume, but most of us also have no way of learning about our own body burdens. The test for PBDEs costs upward of a thousand dollars. Organic pollutants drawn from the environment are not part of any prenatal test. This is probably a good thing, since there is nothing we can do with the knowledge anyway. There is no way to rid our bodies of our chemical burdens, except, sadly, by breastfeeding and passing them along to our infants, whose levels will then be exponentially higher than our own. But it's also worth remembering that we have very little idea about what these levels mean. In some lab tests, mice who receive doses comparable with some American human levels suffer effects like lower intelligence and damaged thyroids, but I've repeatedly been told that the links between chemicals and health problems are almost impossible to prove. It's also worth remembering that the human body is designed to deal with contaminants and has wondrous ways of cleansing itself, to a point.

My levels of PBDEs, it turned out, were smack in the middle of the American average, or 36 parts per billion. This was reassuring in a way, because I wasn't one of those unfortunate statistical outliers, those women and kids who have levels nearing 1,000, for reasons no one understands. But even if I were, it might be insignificant. We simply don't know what these levels mean for ourselves and our babies. And so far, very few Americans have been tested, probably fewer than 300. As one academic told me, it makes more sense to stress yourself out over things you can control, like trans fats and whether your kids' car seats are properly installed.

The critical question for me and for you is whether or not it is safe to breastfeed. Unless you are an Inuit woman (whose diet of harbor seals makes her vulnerable to very high levels of PBDEs) or someone who lives near the site of an industrial accident, the answer is a big yes. This is because the benefits of breastfeeding greatly outweigh the risks, and, frankly, formula is far from pure. Some studies show that breast milk may actually counter the effects of industrial contaminants, even as it increases the levels of those same contaminants. Breastfed children have higher IQs, for example, and your children will need them in a world filled with neurotoxins.

Should we be hysterical? No. Should we be angry? Absolutely. I took that anger to my state legislature, which was considering enacting a ban on PBDEs (several states have done so, including Michigan, Maine, New York, California, and Hawaii). In front of a Health and Human Services subcommittee, I held up a test tube of my breast milk. I waved the pale liquid before the legislators and talked about its miracles and its hazards. The chemical lobby made an impassioned plea about why this legislation was premature. My state chose not to pass the ban, but many others will consider legislation soon.

The European Union banned the two major commercial formulations of PBDEs several years ago. And last year, the EPA reached an agreement with U.S. manufacturers to stop making those same formulations, but existing stockpiles can still be used.

Politically, breastfeeders represent a potentially powerful force. Most American women who breastfeed are college educated and proactive about their children's health. This is the same demographic clamoring for health information about vaccinations, asthma, autism, and behavioral problems in their children. For the antitoxics lobby, these mothers could be a dream, as effective as Mothers Against Drunk Driving. It was not until persistent organic chemicals began appearing in human milk that countries took steps to ban them. It's unfortunate that we have compromised nature's perfect food, but perhaps the time has come for those of us with boobs to try to make them perfect again.

FLORENCE WILLIAMS lives in Montana, where she writes for The New York Times *and* The New York Times Magazine. *She is also a contributing editor to* Outside Magazine.

fish

For some reason there isn't the same amount of black-and-white government information on what is and isn't safe to consume when breastfeeding as when pregnant. Talk to your doctor about specifics, but sushi gets the thumbs up. Continue to stay away from fish high in mercury like swordfish, shark, and tuna (for more on this, see Part 2, "Food").

guzzle

Breastfeeding will not only make you hungry, it will make you thirsty. (One friend said she was so thirsty, she felt like she had ashes in her mouth.) So drink up. A baby consumes many ounces of breast milk a day, and that liquid needs to be replenished. Follow our basic water guidelines (filter and avoid plastic receptacles), and don't fill up on nutritionless, sugary fruit juices. At least now you can return to your favorite juice bar. But don't order the extra vitamins many juice bars push—you're getting plenty from your prenatal (which you should still be taking). Your thirst level will dictate what you need. If you're getting sick of plain old water, what the hell, squeeze in a wedge of lemon.

NURSING TEAS

Tea with fenugreek is thought to promote lactation. It can be made iced in the summer, hot in the winter. For more on herbs, read *Nursing Mother's Herbal* by Sheila Humphrey.

garlic, broccoli, hot peppers

Some breastfeeding literature would have you believe that everything from lentils to cauliflower to chocolate makes for gassy, crying babies. But of course moms from India to Italy eat these supposedly "bad" foods and manage to breastfeed successfully. Your baby might have specific foods that make her fussy, which you'll figure out soon enough and stop eating. Some common offenders include cruciferous veggies like broccoli, cabbage, and brussels sprouts, but these are all so good for you and your baby that you shouldn't cut them out until you have to. In fact, don't give up anything frivolously. Your baby will let you know what bothers her. An unhappy baby can have everything from gas to crying to sleeplessness to skin rashes to diarrhea. If you have a family history of being allergic to cow's milk or wheat, these could be the problem. Ask your doctor to weigh in.

formula

For years there have been only two certified organic formulas for sale in this country: Baby's Only and Horizon Organic. Baby's Only is available at Whole Foods (for other retailers near you: *www.naturesone.com*) but is marketed as toddler formula, not infant formula. (Bring the ingredient list to your pediatrician, who may give it the green light for your infant anyway.) Horizon Organic is available only on the West Coast. This seems like a gaping hole in the organic market to us. Wal-Mart agreed, and recently developed Parents' Choice organic baby formula (*www.parentschoiceformula.com*). There are reasons you want organic formula, and they're the same reasons you choose organic food. Milk-based formulas are derived from cow's milk (of course), so you want a version that wasn't fed nonorganic feed, growth hormones, and antibiotics. Baby's Only also sells a soy-based formula, which is good for babies with milk allergies. There are also nutritional differences between conventional and organic formulas. The oils in the organic versions are traditionally better for you. And the carbohydrate in Baby's Only is certified organic brown rice syrup, as opposed to the corn syrup found in some conventional formulas.

If you're not on the West Coast, don't live near a Wal-Mart, and your doctor doesn't clear you to use toddler formula for your infant, you're going to have to do a lot of nutritional comparisons of conventional formulas. There is one other choice. Some moms take their quest for supplemental milk a step further by using donor milk from human milk banks. Donor milk is pasteurized, and some health care companies will even pay for it. To find out more, go to the Human Milk Banking Association of North America's Web site: *www.hmbana.org*.

Whatever formula you wind up with, keep in mind that powdered formulas are much less sterile than ready-to-feed formulas. If you're mixing a powder with water, make sure to use the purest water possible.

Boobed Out: When Baby Wants More

BY MOON UNIT ZAPPA

Around the fourth month of my baby's life, everyone started harassing me to start giving her "real food," as my mother calls it. (Okay, maybe it was only my mother who was harassing me; she just feels like everyone.) Until then, I had been a breast-milk-only mom, priding myself on the lucky fact that my child never needed a drop of formula. Not that I have anything against formula for other people, it's just that the thought of genetically engineered anything around a fresh human always seemed cruel to me somehow. So, even though my kid showed Dickensian signs of pickpocketing table scraps all too early, we decided to wait until Father's Day, the day after a trip to Hawaii when she would be exactly six months old, to begin the intimidating process of transitioning to solids. I knew that the slight delay would give me a little extra time to research this next phase a little more thoroughly, since the switch to solids seemed impossibly overwhelming to me.

The flight over was a breeze. Mathilda nursed going up and going down for the landing, and a few times in between. But as soon as we deplaned, a blast of tropical heat got to her, and a puking adventure began and escalated by the time I got her into our rental car. When we finally arrived at my ninety-year-old grandmother's place, my child started truly behaving oddly. Abnormally fussy turned into inconsolable, then out-and-out heart-popping, ice-water-bowels hysterical. I more or less wrote it off to a lack of air-conditioning and jet lag and tried to nurse her to sleep like I usually did. She had bled me dry milk-wise, so I decided to pump in the morning, but when her tiny demon eyes flew open at 4 A.M. and stayed open, I got up, too.

On the changing table, I discovered my satanic child had sprouted two previously undetected bottom teeth overnight. Well, that explained something! To be sure, I called my pediatrician to see if colic could come on late, but she assured me it was her new chompers and told me to have a pleasant vacation. I was relieved, thinking the worst was behind us now that the teeth had cut through the gums, but over the course of the day Mathilda was not settling back down into the cute, cuddly baby we had previously grown accustomed to and actually liked. This new fire-breathing baby was trying our patience. To make things stranger, the hand pump I had brought along to save suitcase space was not cutting the pumping dealio. Back on the mainland I was able to extract at least two ounces of liquid gold from each breast, but now on the Island of Sudden Doom I was getting only two ounces between them. To irritate me further, my grandmother (who raised seven children) mentioned that our child seemed hungry to her and asked us when we were going to start giving her real food. (Talk about apples not falling far from the tree.) Indignant, I said, "Breast milk *is* real food and we will start solids once we get back." The truth of the matter was that I was just not ready to say good-bye to the babe-in-arms baby yet, not to mention that the whole process of getting off the boob and into whipping up gourmet infant cuisine intimidated the living daylights out of me.

As our trip wore on, my daughter's moods deteriorated. It was like having a newborn all over again, only worse. She was inconsolable at night, and even more inconsolable during the day. Where once there was some relief at the breast, nursing now seemed to exacerbate her ferocious mania and make her scream louder and longer. Again came my grandmother's rude insistence with mounting frequency that the baby seemed hungry for actual food. "You'll see, with a full belly she'll sleep straight through the night." Dumb bitch. For once I empathized with my mother's usual comments about my grandmother's supposed unsupportive side that I had never noticed before. To top things off, at my usual pumping times I was extracting less and less milk with my stupid hand pump and cursing the fact that I did not pack my enormous Pump In Style so someone else could at least give her a bottle so I could maybe see the goddamn beach for five fucking seconds!

That night I tried to use my hand pump and couldn't extract even half an ounce between my breasts. Something about my total lack of milk in conjunction with my stress level, sleep deprivation, heatstroke, and my grandmother's nasty food comments finally gave me pause to consider maybe something was not just a little wrong with my unusual situation but drastically wrong: Maybe my hand pump had caused my milk supply to vanish and I had unexpectedly weaned my daughter without realizing it and now she was starving to death! Maybe our baby did indeed want solids now, now, *now*!!! Panic set in. The next morning I vowed to start giving her real food. After all, it would be only a few days early. The next day my real ignorance really kicked in.

Until then I had always thought you just started feeding a baby solid foods—you simply bought a jar of baby food, organic, of course, and started. I had no idea that it takes almost two weeks just to get your baby up and running with little more than a tablespoon of cereal and about an eyedropper's worth of pureed fruit. When I called my pediatrician a second time long-distance and she laid out these cold hard facts for me was when hysteria and insanity merged. In Technicolor detail I saw that even if I started solids that minute, it would not make a dent in terms of satisfying my kid's impending death by hunger. Not to mention the small issue of my total grief around the suddenness of losing my nursing baby to the evils of society with its stupid solid foods and the total self-hatred of my asshole body and its flawed mammary glands. All at once I had a fraction of a glimmer of what mothers in starving countries must go through holding their suckling babies to their empty bosoms. I felt sick to my core. At the very least I had to get my milk supply back up and running to some small degree lest I be forced to give my baby—gulp—man-made, factory-fabricated formula!

To make a long story even longer, there were no support resources on that glorious land mass like a lactation consultant or a midwife or doula or hospital that could help me, so I called The Pump Station in L.A. It's amazing what a little bit of knowledge and some human warmth can accomplish. They told me to hit the health food store, drink some water, and get some sleep. Well, the human body is amazing! In the end my baby and my boobies persevered for the three remaining days, thanks to their suggestion of large quantities of Mother's Milk tea, fennel capsules, nursing like a maniac, and eating whole grains like oatmeal and brown rice until I could get back to my deluxe pump at home.

Back home I read books, went online, phoned our pediatrician again, and asked my friends about the amazing evolution from liquid to hearty fare. Now, before I finally pass on the best of what I learned, I must also warn you that if you, too, are waiting to start the "real food" feeding process, don't. See, this phase really does zip by in the blink of an eye. In less than a month our baby got so used to eating the gooey stuff, that all too quickly she desired thicker textures; immediately after that, self-feeding kicked in to high gear. She ate from my spoon for no more than two months before demanding in her nonverbal but very articulate way that she wanted to make her own messes thank you very much. Now, our nine-month-old child lets me sneak in bites of other things only while she is shoveling fistfuls of cottage cheese and Cheerios into her mouth all by herself. So, if you are a control freak who wants to baby your baby for the longest possible time, ironically, start solids sooner. Plus, making your own organic baby food is fun and easy!

It saves you money, it takes hardly any time at all, you know what your baby is eating, it tastes better, and it's a great head start—you can reinvest in your own healthy eating habits by starting your kid out right at the same time. To me, making organic baby food is the next best thing to my cherished breastfeeding to nurture my baby and say "I love you" with food. Have I convinced you? Either way, when you're ready, turn to page 272 in the recipe section to see how to do it.

MOON UNIT ZAPPA is a magazine writer, a stand-up comic, a filmmaker, the author of America the Beautiful, *and a wife and mom. "Boobed Out: When Baby Wants More" © 2006 Moon Unit Zappa. Printed by permission.*

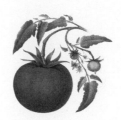

CHAPTER FOURTEEN

home environment

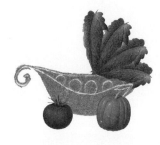

Now that your baby is out of the womb and her home environment is the same as yours, here are some thoughts on staying safe and comfortable.

humidity

If your environment is extremely dry, or wet, humidifiers and dehumidifiers can make sleeping and breathing much easier. The most comfortable rooms tend to have around 50 percent humidity. (You can measure the humidity in the air with a digital hygrometer.) If the air is too dry, it can trigger asthma, or just a plain old stuffy nose that can prevent an infant from sleeping soundly. If you have a baby who sounds like she is snoring when she sleeps, a humidifier will probably help her stop. Be sure not to overhumidify because high humidity can foster the growth of bacteria and allergy-causing mold. You have to weigh the risks and benefits. Be sure to limit the potential spread of bacteria that can grow in the machine by carefully following the cleaning guidelines. Obviously use white vinegar instead of bleach or any of the other solutions sold with your machine. A large selection of humidifiers and dehumidifiers is available at *www.allergybuyersclub.com*.

THE HYGIENE HYPOTHESIS

Don't worry so much about germs. In the late nineties, a German doctor named Erika Von Mutius came up with a theory called "The Hygiene Hypothesis" that says that in order for your child to develop a competent immune system, she actually needs to interact with some germs and allergens. Von Mutius proposes that without enough exposure to microbes, a baby's immune system can be negatively affected. Studies in Japan and Germany have found that babies exposed to other babies have stronger immune systems and fewer allergies than those who spent most of their time at home alone in antiseptic environments. Other studies have found that adults raised on farms were less likely to develop allergies, and that young children exposed to older siblings at home, and those who attend day care, have a lower risk of allergies and asthma. A study done in Sweden and Estonia found that babies raised in sterile hospital environments experienced a sixfold increase in allergies. The bottom line? Some germs are good for you. This doesn't mean you shouldn't wash your hands before picking up your newborn. It just means you can relax a little about the world being a filthy place to grow up. Or, as Deirdre's mother would say: "You need to eat a pound of dirt before you die."

organic tips for inducing sleep

The following tricks have been collected from friends who have used them to get seemingly inconsolable babies to sleep:

White noise—Make your own white noise with fans, vacuum cleaners, portable vacuums, electric toothbrushes, bathroom fans, electric razors, or, to save electricity, recordings of them. Fish tanks that bubble, loud clocks, and metronomes have also worked. Tape-record the sound of a shower or water running from a faucet. The repetitive monotony of these noises mimics the sounds of the womb and can soothe a baby for whom a silent room might feel unnaturally quiet.

Music—If you don't have the energy to sing your baby to sleep, tape yourself singing and press "play" instead. If you can't stand singing, test-run some other music and discover what your baby finds relaxing.

Taped crying—A recording of your baby's own crying, or a recording of another baby crying, can be disconcerting enough to interrupt an upset baby long enough for her to fall asleep.

Dark room—Sounds obvious, but a completely dark room can be less distracting.

The birth ball—Recycle your old birthing ball and use it the way you would a glider. Your baby will love the bouncing, the same way she seems to love anything that forces you to get off the couch and work for her.

Drive—When worse comes to worst, or even before, a trip around the block in the car is often just what a baby needs to fall asleep.

Movement—As long as the baby is safely buckled in, swings and vibrating bouncy seats can be a great way to doze off. Similarly, a sling, Björn, or stroller can do the trick.

washing clothes

Be sure to use the least toxic (fragrance-free) detergents possible, and, of course, always avoid chlorine-based bleaches. Natural laundry detergents (which often contain borax), and natural bleaches are available (more and more often right in your grocery store) from brands like Ecover and Seventh Generation, as well as the Web sites below. (While we're on the subject of clothes, take whatever hand-me-downs are offered, and don't be shy about asking for more. Most people are thrilled for the chance to recycle.)

www.ecover.com
www.vermontsoap.com
www.greenfeet.com
www.naturallyyoursclean.com
www.seventhgeneration.com
www.oxyboost.com

bottles

Whether you're pumping or using formula, you can't take the safety of your bottles for granted. Most bottles are plastic, but unlike disposable water bottles, they're used over and over, heated to clean and frozen for storing milk. Wear and tear makes them more likely to leach their chemicals. Polycarbonate (#7) is commonly used for baby bottles, and contains bisphenol-A, a hormone-disrupting chemical. PVC can also be found in bottles as well as nipples, and should be avoided. Not all bottles are labeled with the kind of plastic they're made out of, so do what we do: buy glass bottles. They were good enough for generations before us. Evenflo makes four-ouncers, which are easiest for small babies to hold, and the glass is shatter resistant. If you have to use plastic, look for decoration-free bottles made from plastic #2 or #5. But be careful, don't heat the milk while it's in the plastic bottles. Avoid disposable bottle systems with plastic bags attached. Don't forget about bacteria, either; it grows in the scratches. As soon as your bottle looks worn, throw it away. And recycle glass bottles the minute you spy a chip. For more information, look up the baby bottle product report at *www.thegreenguide.com.*

nipples and pacifiers

Most bottle nipples and pacifiers are made of either rubber or silicone. If you buy glass bottles, they come with traditional latex nipples. Latex allergies are on the rise, so much so that balloons are routinely banned in hospital maternity wards. We suggest replacing latex nipples as well as rubber ones (which are suspected to release carcinogens) with safer, silicone versions. As with bottles, always inspect nipples for cracks and tears, which could be breeding grounds for bacteria. Pacifiers—love them or hate them—can sometimes contain PVC. Clearly you don't want your child sucking on that. Use silicone here as well.

sterilization

All bottles, nipples, and pacifiers should be sterilized before their first use. Dishwashers that heat water up to 180 degrees F are sufficient. Try to use the least harsh detergents and soaps you can find. We have dishwasher-less friends who either use steam sterilizers or boil bottles on their stoves.

pumps

When it comes to pumping your milk, there's no way around plastic—the tubing, shields, and receptacles are all made out of it. Women vary on the pumps they like. Some moms can make a hand pump work, and others rent industrial-sized versions. The most common choice is an electric home pump that costs a few hundred dollars. Sharing these pumps with friends is controversial. Medela, a manufacturer of one of the most popular home pumps, calls them "personal use" products, like toothbrushes. The government also comes out against sharing. Unlike industrial pumps, home versions aren't made with a closed system, so milk can back up into the motor. You can boil or buy new parts, but there is ultimately no way to sterilize the motor. In the unlikely event that milk backed up into the motor before the pump was given to you, disease and bacteria could still be living in there and could possibly harm your baby. For this reason, we don't advocate buying a used personal-use pump off eBay or Craig's List, or taking a hand-me-down.

milk storage

Plastic seems to be the most common receptacle available for storing breast milk. Many companies sell plastic storage bags specifically to go in the fridge and freezer, but we opt for glass here, too. You can freeze directly in glass bottles or in freezer-safe glass jars. Just don't fill either to the top, so there is room for the liquid to expand. Besides avoiding leaching plastic, there is some speculation in the lactation consultant community that breast milk nutrients cling to plastic but not to glass, which seems like a big waste of valuable nourishment.

The Nontoxic Nursery

BY JULIE TORRES MOSKOVITZ

As I prepare construction on my eighteen-month-old son's room in our loft in an old factory building, I contemplate what level of eco-friendly and organic to aim for. My son confronts all types of toxic materials every day in our neighborhood. We live in Williamsburg, Brooklyn, in a mixed-use zone where industry is side by side with residential living, so we are probably exposed to more hazardous chemicals in our air than the average suburban dweller. Sometimes I contemplate moving out of the city, escaping to a cleaner environment. However, I do not allow myself to fixate on this daydream because in the end I know that unsafe materials are found everywhere and there is no use trying to run away. Instead, I've decided to embrace the choice we've made to stay here and raise a child. There are positives to being in an old factory building; aside from the high ceilings and great views, our space is drafty, which to me indicates that we have an air exchange. This assures me that we are not living in a "sick air" building.

I begin my journey into creating a room for my precious baby boy just as I created a safe haven for him in my womb. My choice in materials and paints for my son's room has evolved and expanded over time. I know this from the research that I have collected for my architecture practice, Fabrica 718, which specializes in sustainable design. Thanks to the demands of forward-looking clients, I've found many environmentally friendly products in recent years. These products fit into several categories: those made from recycled materials, those that promote conservation of the environment, and those that provide a safer, cleaner home environment. I've researched many eco-materials in an effort to determine which category they fall into, and to figure out whether it's truly a "green" material or if a company is just profiteering from the new eco-friendly trend. My clients are often drawn to wood materials like OSB (oriented strand board) and a derivative product called COR, which are good in terms of the greater environment because they use upward of 70 percent of a tree versus solid wood products that use only 40 percent. But they are made with toxic glues and therefore emit VOCs. There are also companies that use recycled plastic, but add to it a resin. This creates a new, unrecyclable material. Once these plastic resin materials have lived their useful life, they will be sent to the landfill and there they will never degrade and return to the earth.

On top of deciphering product literature to determine if something is actually a "green" material, there's the obstacle of finding a contractor who is willing to use it. I have faced resistance from contractors who automatically want to charge a higher price for eco-friendly materials because of the extra effort they predict they will need to spend to find and work with something that varies from the standard. I always do the background research on availability and pricing so that I am prepared to help the contractor. Calling ahead of time to determine the correct distributor to order from is critical, because otherwise your project can be held up waiting for these specialty materials. I've also discovered that a lot of environmental products are frequently discontinued or distributors suddenly stop carrying them. Although "green" design has grown in popularity, business can be slow. For example, I was planning on using Dow's Woodstalk, a compressed wheatgrass for the bed frame for my son's bed. I have used Woodstalk on many projects. A four-by-eight-foot sheet, three-quarter-inch-thick, costs less than an average piece of three-quarter-inch thick plywood. However, I recently learned that Woodstalk has just been discontinued. Fortunately, I have found several similar products on the market.

In choosing where to locate my son's room within our open loft space, I decided that encompassing a large window was a good idea. Although babies need dark spaces to take naps in during the day, the value of good ventilation outweighs the need for darkness. For his furniture, I will use several products that I have used in other architecture projects. I recently designed a bar in New York City's East Village, where the client insisted on using a compressed wheatgrass board for the bar and seating areas. This material has held up very well with high traffic and use. Primeboard premium wheatboard is now the most readily available alternative to Dow's Woodstalk. I will either leave this wheatgrass board in its natural color, using only a water-based sealer, or choose a nontoxic, semi-gloss paint finish for it. Safecoat (www.safecoatpaint.com) and Best Paint (www.bestpaintco.com) offer beautiful, rich color options. For a clear, satin sealer I'll buy AFM Natural's Safecoat Polyureseal (www.afmsafecoat.com). Titebond (www.titebond.com) has a line of safe, water-based wood glue I will use to construct the furniture.

For building my son's bed frame and bookshelving, I am planning on using a compressed wood board that has no formaldehyde: Medite II by SierraPine (www.sierrapine.

com). I will stain it with one of the eight Safecoat DuroStains available by AFM Naturals. His mattress will be organic and I may opt for the twin size (39"W × 75"L) so that it will last longer than the smaller toddler size (28"W × 52"L).

For painting the walls of his room, I have several safe options that come in a wide range of colors. I'll use the eggshell finish by AFM Safe Coat or possibly the more muted colors offered by Milk Paint (*www.milkpaint.com*). In the past I have used Benjamin Moore's Eco Spec paint, which comes in hundreds of colors and is more readily available than these paints. However, Benjamin Moore does not offer the saturated colors in its Eco Spec line. Adding fun colors to a child's bedroom walls is an easy and cost-effective way to distinguish it and make it feel like his or her own, unique place. My architecture partner took this idea one step further by painting an abstract, colorful mural on one wall in her daughter's room.

And I will not carpet the room. Since asthma is a concern for city dwellers, I want to be sure that my son's room is dust-free, which means avoiding wall-to-wall carpeting. To keep things cozy, we may have a small area rug of natural grass or a biodegradable, non-toxic one by manufacturers such as Earthweave Carpet Mills, Inc. (*www.earthweave.com*) or Colin Campbell & Sons (*www.naturescarpet.com*).

Being eco-friendly should never feel like you are compromising aesthetically. New ideas can develop from the limitations of green product availability. Details such as differently sized niches built into the walls of the room can offer many options for storing toys and books in interesting ways. This is a simple detail to add to your child's room that doesn't involve introducing toxic or harmful materials to his or her room. The best architectural feature in my son's room won't be organic or eco-friendly but special just the same: a small access way into our bedroom so that he can feel free to come and jump in bed with us.

Julie Torres Moskovitz is an architect in New York City who focuses on green design. She is working on a line of sustainable children's furniture, available at www.fabrica718.com.

diapers

Cloth or disposable? We used to think this was a total no-brainer. Why would you throw anything in a landfill if there was an alternative? The EPA statistics on how many diapers a year Americans toss into landfills (18 billion in 1990) are as depressing as it gets. Plus, babies in cloth diapers are said to be more likely to potty train earlier than disposable diaper babies (a baby who is never wet is less likely to give up wearing her diapers). But then we researched what it takes diaper services to clean cloth diapers: lots of extremely hot water and lots and lots of chlorine bleach. And that didn't sound appealing in the least, for the baby's tender skin or for the dioxin levels in the environment (dioxin is the carcinogenic byproduct of chlorine bleaching; see page 32). Plus, you never know what was in the industrial washing machine before your baby's diapers.

If you can wash cloth diapers at home using chlorine alternatives in a washing machine with really hot water, great. Your choice is made. This is an inexpensive (if time-consuming) way of dealing with the diapering dilemma. Sure, you'll use a lot of water, but so do the cloth diaper delivery services, and the manufacturers of disposable diapers. Just try to find diaper covers that aren't plastic or don't contain plastic, especially PVC. There are plenty of (sometimes organic) cotton and wool versions available.

If you aren't set up to wash cloth diapers at home, conventional disposable diapers aren't a good option. One widely quoted study (published in Archives of Environmental Health and conducted by Anderson Laboratories back in 1999) found mice exposed to VOC chemicals emitted by conventional disposables had asthmalike reactions. They also contain chlorine and have high-tech chemical gel cores that activate when your baby pees to "lock in moisture." The Children's Health Environmental Coalition says this absorbent material—sodium polyacrylate—could cause respiratory and skin irritations in occupational settings (where exposure is higher than with diaper use). We wonder how safe can that much chemical activity that close to a baby's genitals be twenty-four hours a day?

The other choice is to use environmentally friendly disposable diapers like Tushies. They're a cotton-blend diaper made with chlorine-free wood pulp that contains no chemicals or gels. (Some other brands of "environmental" disposables do use gel if you read the fine print.) Tushies can be found at Whole Foods, or can be delivered to your door via UPS (*www.tushies.com*). They're more expensive than conventional diapers, and without the lock-in mechanism you'll have to change them more often. They're also still disposable, chlorine or no chlorine. There is no such thing as a biodegradable diaper. Still, alternative disposables use less material than conventional ones.

Each diapering option—cloth or disposable—has its drawbacks. If you have free time on your hands, you could train your baby to go diaperless. Invest in a copy of Ingrid Bauer's *Diaper Free! The Gentle Wisdom of Natural Infant Hygiene.*

diaper resources

The Children's Health Environmental Coalition (*www.checnet.org*) estimates a baby goes through an average of 8,000 diapers from birth to toilet training. For more information on the 8,000 your infant will go through:

- *www.diaperjungle.com*
- *www.babynaturale.com*
- *www.seventhgeneration.com*
- *www.tushies.com*
- *www.naty.se*
- *www.diapernet.org* (The National Association of Diaper Services)

The Junk in My Trunk

BY CHRISTIE MELLOR

I was determined to use cloth diapers, and to be the most environmentally friendly mommy I could be, so I signed up with a diaper service, those nice people who drive around L.A. in natural-gas-powered trucks and recycle their water. (A process I didn't want to know too much about.) Also, we lived in a one-bedroom apartment with no washing machine or dryer, which may have been a factor in my decision to use the diaper service, as opposed to spending every waking hour of my life washing diapers in the kitchen sink.

We used to drive from Los Angeles to San Francisco fairly often for the first five months of my son's life; he was only a few days old when we found out my mother had pancreatic cancer, and my sisters and I would convene on a regular basis to see her, and to help out my dad and the hospice people. For our first big trip there, I brought extra diapers. About two weeks' worth. So imagine, if you will, two weeks' worth of fermenting, festering baby waste piling up in the corner of the room. It's not half as cute or sweet-smelling as you might think.

When we were packing up to go back to Los Angeles, I just remember lugging giant, heavy garbage bags full of wet, stinking, poopy diapers out to the trunk of the car, and squeezing them in on top of our luggage, and opening the trunk back in L.A. and having to hold our breath, and putting the bags out on the front stoop for the long-suffering Tidee Didee man.

Although the feeling of personal virtue lasted for quite a while, I decided that disposable diapers, if only for trips and such, wouldn't necessarily be the death of the planet. I continued to faithfully use cloth diapers but decided that sometimes you have to find ways to make your life not such a living hell. I asked the landfill gods to forgive me and started taking disposables on our subsequent trips. I also allowed us one disposable diaper a night, which helped the baby sleep longer, and hence, helped me get more sleep. It seemed like a fair compromise.

CHRISTIE MELLOR is a writer in L.A. and the author of The Three Martini Playdate: A Practical Guide to Happy Parenting.

work environment

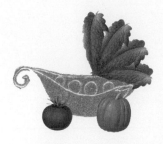

the cafeteria

If you're newly back at work, you're probably spending all your downtime furiously pumping in a locked office instead of enjoying leisurely lunches at the most organic restaurant you can find. If your office has a cafeteria, it's worth putting in a request for some basic organic items like cheese, fruit, eggs, whole-wheat bread, and lettuce. If you can't force organic food on your caterer, just apply the same ideas about eating you did during pregnancy: whole foods are always best. Stay away from typical lunchtime food like deli meats, which are full of nitrates, hormones, and antibiotics. If you've got a salad bar, supplement your lettuce with the least contaminated vegetables, like avocados, broccoli, sweet corn, onions, cauliflower, and sweet peas. Same goes for fruit—look for kiwi, bananas, mangoes, papaya, and pineapple. Probably none of these will be local or even in season—it's a cafeteria after all. If you're craving hot food, pick something vegetarian like a veggie burger, or vegetarian lasagna or another pasta.

Milking It: A Survival Guide to Pumping at Work and Working at Home

BY TERRI KURTZBERG

I keep reading in baby magazines about companies that have "lactation rooms" equipped with couches, electrical outlets in convenient places, and, of course, soft lighting and plenty of privacy. I know of nobody, however, who has actually seen one of these with her own eyes, so I am starting to think that they are one of our generation's urban legends, an oasis we can all picture but never quite reach in reality. Instead, pumping breast milk at work is fraught with its challenges.

I know I'm not alone in my experience through conversations with my girlfriends. One told me of how she went back to her car to pump (and hoped that nobody left early that day). Another hung a Do Not Enter sign on the bottom of a set of stairs to a loft, since the entire office she worked in was visible on the main floor. A third told me about having to explain to her male coworkers that when her office door was closed, it meant that she was available neither to answer the door nor to pick up the phone (which they routinely tried two minutes later).

My own situation caused me to feel a little like Fonzie from *Happy Days;* remember the way he used to refer to the men's room as his "office"? I'm a professor at Rutgers University, and my classes the semester after my baby was born happened to be scheduled in a different building from my office, so returning to the privacy of my office was not an option. Instead, the first day of class found me, during break, scrambling from bathroom to bathroom trying to find an appropriate setup. My class was on the second floor of a three-story building. I decided to try going upstairs to the third-floor ladies' room, thinking that even if our closest bathroom was busy, the students would be less likely to climb the stairs (or wait for the ancient elevator) to find another one. Best-laid plans: the third-floor ladies' room had no electrical outlet. I scrambled back down to the first-floor bathroom. There, at last, was an outlet next to a high shelf. This meant I would need to stand while I pumped, not really relaxing but far better than having to go all seven hours without nursing relief. After I got all hooked up to pump both sides at once, I turned on the switch, and nothing happened. Panic. Luckily, before I totally melted down, I tried resetting the outlet and it worked. Whew.

For the most part, my hideaway was relatively private, but at least once per pumping "session" someone would walk in and see me. At first, I hated these interruptions, as there are rarely more exposed moments to be found than being hooked up to a breast pump. However, little by little I began to appreciate the pump for the conversation-starter that it was. First day: In walked one of my students, who promptly asked me how the baby was doing and encouraged my activities. Another memorable time was the day one of the female janitorial staff came into the room to clean while I was pumping. The woman, maybe sixty years old and from another country, barely spoke English. She took a look at me and my apparatus, pointed, and asked, "Baby?" I agreed, and she took a closer look at the machine. "Wow" was what she had to offer. Then, in halting English, she communicated perfectly: "In my day . . ." I agreed again, and commented on how great it was to have an electric pump to do the work for you.

Pumping at work is hard, but I got an appreciation for the universality of breastfeeding through my encounters, week after week, with people in the ladies' room on campus. It was one of the most significant senses of community that I have ever experienced, much to my surprise.

But as hard as pumping at work is, working at home presents its own set of challenges. People told me before I had my baby that working from home is easier at the beginning, when the baby is willing to just sleep or play quietly in a cradle while you work. Not my baby. I had a hold-me-all-the-time baby from day 1, and an I-know-who-Mom-is-and-who-isn't baby from about six weeks on. This made my work-at-home days something of a challenge. Now, eight months into the game, I look back and realize that I've developed a few strategies along the way for meeting my baby's needs and accomplishing my own professional goals as well. Mostly, the insights ended up being adaptations of the advice you hear from everyone.

#1: Work when the baby sleeps. This is sound advice, except at the very beginning when, of course, you need to try to sleep when the baby sleeps. However, with a few exceptions—like when she will fall asleep in her swing or I have the luxury of a babysitter who will take her out in her carriage for her nap—Jillian likes to sleep on my lap. I suppose I could have forced the issue and worked her toward a willingness to nap in her crib, but instead I found two other solutions. The first is a fully functional, and entirely portable, office setup. I have a laptop and a wireless network setup in the house. I have a stack table and close enough proximity to an outlet. And I have a list of things in my head that I try not to sit down without: the portable phone, a glass of water and sometimes a snack, TV remotes, reading material, a Binky for the baby, and, of course, the computer. While Jillian nurses and then snoozes, I get some of my most productive thinking time in. In fact, she's sleeping on my lap as I write this. This system, though it seems obvious now, was hard fought and won, nearly at the cost of our marital harmony. When I was newer to all of this, I would scurry to my spot on the couch with the baby as soon as she cried in hunger, and then would find myself trapped without any of the things I needed to make good use of that time for myself (translation: in addition to not being able to work productively, I was bored). My husband (when he was home with us) was stretched to the limits of his patience by my requests for the same six items about twelve times a day, until I truly got the hang of setting myself up ahead of time. We call the stack table my "station" now, and both of us know to put things back there when they walk off. Occasionally, I can also use the sling, which works less reliably but sometimes will keep Jillian sleeping for hours strapped to my body while I am totally free to walk around the house or sit down and work.

#2: Delegate or put off what doesn't really need doing. Working at home means working in an environment full of distractions. It also means an endless to-do list of laundry, cleaning, house chores, baby-care tasks, and, of course, work. It's too easy to let work fall to the bottom of the list. I'm sure some people can do it all without any help, but I couldn't. One of the insights for me was not that I should hire in some help, but rather what I should get help with. Our babysitter, Sarah, is truly a Renaissance woman, and if she were a Girl Scout, I'm sure she would be eligible for any one of about ten different merit badges. She watches the baby, of course, but when Jillian is nursing or sleeping, Sarah does a million other things for us. Not just grocery shopping and cooking, although those are obviously valuable, but also help with all of the things that create stresses in our household. Often this means doing jobs my husband doesn't have time for anymore, like filing or tying up the recycling. She reorganizes our closets. She folds up leftover shopping bags. She records my students' grades in the spreadsheet when I'm done reading papers. And, most important, she is willing to walk for miles to let the baby sleep in the carriage. I find I need to ask myself all the time, "What are the jobs I would rather do than be working?" and most of those go to Sarah, which frees up my mind and my time for my work.

#3: Create tasks with reasonable time demands. Gone are the days when I could sit and work on a paper or project for several days with anything like true immersion. One of the real insights that I have found is the need to be able to break down every task into small units. This is true not just for my job, but also for anything else I try to accomplish in the house. Everybody knows that the second you start putting the wash in the dryer, the baby will suddenly, and simultaneously, need to eat and to be changed. It took me a long time to come to grips with the lack of finishing anything, but when I was finally able to let go of that bottom-line sense of accomplishment and see each step as a separate project, it really freed me up to get more done and feel better about it all.

I know I'm not done figuring out how to work from home. Jillian is getting more savvy, and at this point she knows that when either my husband or I take her into our home office and walk toward the computer, we are likely to have our attention drawn away from her for long minutes, so she preemptively cries before we even sit down. I'm also planning on installing doors on that room to make sure that I can separate from the household activity, once that starts to become a problem. I love my work-at-home days in spite of all the hoops I need to jump through to make them work. And so going forward, I know that whenever new problems arise, there'll be a new answer.

TERRI KURTZBERG is an assistant professor of organizational behavior at the Rutgers Business School in New Jersey.

separation anxiety

When to return to work after having a baby is obviously an extremely personal choice, but here are a few things to think about when deciding: For one thing, realize that you might not be able to predict how you're going to feel about leaving the new love of your life until the moment you kiss her good-bye, so don't feel bad if you decide to change your mind. You might not have the financial freedom to not work, but just because you've spent months lining up a day care/nanny/babysitting situation you're happy with doesn't mean you have to stick to it.

If you talked to your boss before you left for maternity leave about working from home part-time after the baby, follow up on it when you return. Don't feel guilty about having these conversations. You'll probably be twice as productive without office politics to deal with anyway.

Another idea to consider is going back to work part-time for less money. If you think you can't afford to, think about what you might give up so that you could. A new baby isn't another addition to a list of things you spend money on, but an opportunity to rethink everything in your life (including what you spend money on). The sooner you stop thinking about your child as something that fits into one of the many time slots of which your day is divided, the easier it will be for you to accept the fact that you don't have the time to do as many of the things you used to take for granted.

Finally, and this is a no-brainer, talk to lots of people. If you're not hearing what you want, talk to more people. Once you have a child, your world expands, and you'll probably notice you're more open than you used to be. You're literally invested in the world in a way you've never experienced. You want to help people, and you want them to help you. But when it comes to balancing motherhood and work, women still aren't sure exactly what's expected. There's still no right answer and probably never will be, because there aren't enough hours in the day to be with your child and work as much as you might want or need to. We're guilty if we work too much, or too little, and some of that guilt is the direct result of criticism (real or perceived) from other moms. Keep talking to people until you find the support you need to help you make a decision you're comfortable with.

pumping industriously

To hear some women tell it, an industrial pump is to a home pump as a Lexus is to a skateboard. They say the milk flows effortlessly from your breast, the pump purrs quietly, and it is way faster. We know a number of women who fed their babies for as long as they wanted to with home or individual hand pumps, but industrial pumps are something you might also consider if you're not the only one with a newborn at home.

Industrial pumps can be rented (for around $50 a month from hospitals or specialty lactation boutiques) and left in your office for you and any number of women to use. Even if you split the cost with only one other woman, you could end up saving more money than if you bought a portable electric pump for a few hundred bucks. Industrial pumps are built to be shared, with a closed system. This means milk can't back up into the motor, and there is no risk of milk contamination. The trickiest part of sharing an industrial pump at work will probably be working out the schedule of who uses it when.

day care

You've worked hard to create a pure environment for your child at home, so keep in mind that a group day care situation is likely to be a much more conventional environment than your living room. (If you can't find a day care that you like, you can also look into doing a nanny share with a like-minded friend.) When considering different day cares, here are some questions to keep in mind:

- What is the ratio of caretakers to babies?
- Can the infant nap when she wants, or does she have to nap in a group?
- What kind of mattress is your child going to be sleeping on? If PVC-covered, would they be open to your bringing your own organic or wool cover for it?
- What kind of ventilation is there? Will the windows be open?
- Is there a wall-to-wall carpet?
- Will the staff carry your baby in a sling you provide?
- If you use cloth diapers, will they use them, too?
- Are they willing to feed the baby your pumped milk?
- For formula users, is the facility's water filtered?

Galley Slave: My Ill-Timed Maternity Leave

BY SUSAN BURTON

For me, organic was a given; I grew up in Boulder, Colorado, popping straws into soy-milk drink boxes and taking down phone messages from my mother's friends about protesting the chemical plant. So when I got pregnant, I focused less on what was organic and more on what was "natural": that was the shorthand I used in my brain. It was natural to take long walks, but maybe not to go running. It was natural to eat steak instead of taking iron supplements. It was natural not to want the epidural. And it was natural to take time off after the baby was born. Unfortunately, this was looking like a problem.

I was writing a book. It was a good book to be writing while pregnant: Pretty much all I had to do was sit at my computer and talk on the phone and write. I didn't have to travel, not even in the morning, except for the time I failed the glucose screen and had to take the long test at a lab downtown. Luckily the results were good: I didn't have gestational diabetes, meaning I could continue drinking hot chocolate and feeling the baby kick, watching the pages pile up and my stomach grow, imagining the languorous spring and summer months we'd spend together, my son and I, strolling in the park and sitting in coffee shops, with my book's publication to look forward to in the fall. Of course, I had to finish writing the book first, but that wouldn't be a problem: I was working fast; I had a schedule.

But time was tight: every day counted so much, it mattered whenever I lost even one or two. Like when my grandmother visited over Thanksgiving, and she and my mother and sister and I all went shopping for the nursery. "I don't know your colors, but I'd love to get you this," my grandmother said, cupping her hand around a green lamp shaped like a dragonfly. "Oh, your grandfather would have been so happy," she'd cried when we'd returned from the twenty-week ultrasound with the news that the baby was a boy. I'd lost those days for the book, but how could I have changed that? Those days mattered, and I wouldn't have wanted them any other way.

So it went with other things, and so it was that I found myself, four days overdue, sitting at my computer, the one expectant mother who actually wanted to stay pregnant just a little longer, so she could get just a little more work done. It was a scenario befitting my worst self: the one who was always grumpy on summer weekends because she needed to get back to the city to finish something, the one who made reporting phone calls from the dark hotel room in Montana while her husband fished alone under brilliant sun. It had been an article of faith that the one time in my life I actually wouldn't work, wouldn't do anything at all, except be with the baby, or, when the baby was sleeping, read books about the baby, was in the months immediately after the baby was born. There was a term for this: *maternity leave.* It was something regular people did, all over the world. Something inside me dropped; there was warmth, and my water. I looked away from my computer, down at my corduroy pants, darkening. Maternity leave: It was natural. And it was not to be.

Nick, our tiny, amazing Nick, was born on a Tuesday evening in April. We came home from the hospital on Thursday, and on Saturday I sent my first work e-mail. At our child-birth class, they'd told you to sleep when the baby did. That obviously was not going to happen. I'd nurse, and Nick would get woozy, and we'd swaddle him and put him in the bassinet. Then I'd go to my desk and work until he cried. I'd nurse again, maybe on the couch, which my mother had covered with receiving blankets. My husband, Mike, would slip a pillow under my arm for support, like the lactation consultant had suggested at the hospital. I'd watch Nick, our tender baby creature, and then I'd hand him to Mike and return to my screen.

I wasn't writing new chapters: It wasn't as bad as that. I was reading the manuscript and making changes to prepare it for typesetting. The book had been written quickly—there were two of us working on it, me and my coauthor, an Afghan-American teenager whom the story was about—and, to my mind, it was a mess. I was drawing lines and arrows and penciling in new paragraphs. I was fact-checking, too, the whole entire 331-page thing. The work was tedious and time-consuming, and it was always hovering. On a crisp day we took Nick to his one-week pediatrician's appointment and, afterward, we walked through the park, along the same path I had covered so many times with him inside. I was so happy, I was trembling. Mike took a picture of me in front of red tulips. Then we came home and I returned a call from the publishing house's lawyer, who wanted me to fax things. It kept on like this: a series of deflations that soon felt crushing.

My OB's office liked to see first-time mothers after two weeks. I sat there, on the high table, the paper crinkling underneath. I had been a nervous patient, but the baby had been born and he had turned out okay. "See?" my doctor said. "All those things you worried about and he's perfect." How was I doing, she wondered. Well, sleep-deprived, but that was fine. The one problem was that I had to finish this book. "You're working?" my doctor said. "Can't you take a break?" She sounded concerned, a way she'd never sounded before, even when I'd had worrisome ultrasounds. My whole pregnancy, I'd felt less worthy than the other women I saw in the doctor's office. They unbuttoned blazers and checked messages while they waited for their turn. I came in jeans and read *Parents*. My doctor was my own age, maybe one or two years older; I'd seen the Northwestern diplomas on her wall. She must think I'm stupid, I figured, or wealthy. I never showed up in office clothes; I was never in a rush. "You work at home, right?" she'd checked once, and I answered yes, vigorously, conveying my industriousness. Still, I was embarrassed about my luck. That I could work from home, that it was little trouble for me to be pregnant. But now, just two weeks later, it was the opposite. Before I'd felt ashamed for having it too easy; now I felt pathetic for not having planned better, for having made it too hard.

In books I read about short leaves, but there was nothing about no leave, or a leave at the wrong time. I looked for more reassurance online, where I found a story about Bonnie Fuller, the tyrannical celebrity-magazine boss, who'd approved page proofs from the maternity ward. Needless to say, this was not the soothing anecdote I'd been seeking, especially given that I read my manuscript while Nick nursed. I piled the pages next to me on the bed and stretched to reach them with my mechanical pencil. The lead kept snapping, which terrified me. I'd check for it in the folds of Nick's gown. Sometimes I had my laptop beside me, too. I got e-mails from a neighborhood mother's group I'd signed up for. They were meeting at the tot lot, or under a tree in the park, or at the coffee shop on a day that it rained. I'd imagine them together, bouncing their newborns on their laps, radiating wonder from this baby-globe of new motherhood that they were completely inside. I was only a couple weeks behind, but it already felt too late to join them there.

On the weekends Mike and I would get coffee and muffins and sit on a bench in the park. A group of elderly Asian women did qigong; we watched them stretch and rolled the stroller in place, lulling Nick to sleep. We'd be sitting there together on a bench in the park, our new little family, and I'd be thinking about Afghanistan. I'd be looking at the green expanse and thinking of opium fields in Afghanistan, and if we had included the line about there being one across from the U.S. base, and if so, did we have a second source that there really was opium there.

I'd hoped that maybe the book wouldn't matter so much once the baby was born. It was disconcerting to still feel the same. I was disappointed that the baby hadn't made everything else in my life seem minuscule. When you have a baby, everyone tells you that your life will never be the same; unfortunately, some of the parts you might like to change don't.

I did one round of changes, and then another, on galley proofs. I made so many changes that my editor called to tell me that my amount of changes was "not normal." We would be charged for the extra production work; it would come out of our royalties. I didn't care; the book was done. I bounced Nick in his baby chair. He was six weeks old. Six weeks: Now it doesn't sound like that long. But the weeks were so dense, so chaotic, that they seemed to add up to more than they were.

Now that the book was done, being a mother was finally beginning. Nick and I had our days together. I bumped his stroller into Starbucks for iced coffee; I wheeled him one-handed on the way up to the park. He sat in his baby chair and watched while I emptied the dishwasher, folded laundry. Of course, it wasn't perfect: It took a while to rid my mind of book thoughts. And Nick cried, piercingly, in public places, which made me self-conscious. But the pages of the book were, at last, in neat, untouched piles! We dismantled my desk and moved all my Afghanistan books into our bedroom. We hung a gingham curtain on the window and expanded Nick's bassinet into a crib, and there it was: the office had become a nursery.

It wasn't long before the mothers of my baby generation were resuming their regular lives. It took me a while to feel ready. When I did return to work, I did so part-time. Getting back into it was hard. Sometimes it seemed I was advancing as Nick did: building strength, incrementally, to roll and sit and crawl. And, of course, staring into my old little laptop at a new desktop photo of Nick, I asked myself: What is natural? Shouldn't I be home with him instead of here, doing this? But it turned out that this new stuff wasn't much like a pesticide: You couldn't decide whether it was natural based on whether it was manufactured in a lab or not. It would take time to figure out, and I might always feel out of sync. Maybe everyone felt that way; I didn't know. What I knew for sure was natural was my fierce love for Nick. Nick, who'd begun smiling, laughing, growing teeth, eating Cheerios, throwing Cheerios, babbling, commando crawling, and pulling his own books down off the shelves.

SUSAN BURTON *is a contributing editor of* This American Life *and a former editor of* Harper's. *She is the coauthor of* Come Back to Afghanistan: A California Teenager's Story.

CHAPTER FIFTEEN

wellness

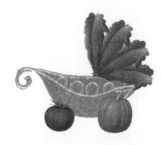

why breastfeed?

Some breastfeeding thoughts from Sandra Steingraber, Ph.D., mother, biologist, and CHEC Advisory Board member. The following excerpt was adapted by the Children's Health Environmental Coalition (*www.checnet.org*) from Steingraber's book *Having Faith: An Ecologist's Journey to Motherhood*.

Stories in the media about the chemical contamination of human milk have made many mothers wonder if bottle-feeding might be an equally healthy alternative to breastfeeding. It is not. The choice is very clear: *Your own breast milk is, hands down, the best food for your baby—far better than its inferior pretender infant formula.* This is the conclusion I reached after more than two years of studying the data on the chemical contamination of breast milk. It's why I nursed Faith for more than two years.

Let's first look at the benefits breast milk offers your baby. Then we'll examine the contamination issue. Breast milk is not just food. It is also medicine. It swarms with antibodies and white blood cells drawn from your own body. By drinking it, your infant comes to share your immune system. And benefits mightily from it. Breastfed infants have lower rates of hospitalization and death. They develop fewer respiratory infections, gastrointestinal infections, urinary tract infections, ear infections, and meningitis. They succumb less often from Sudden Infant Death Syndrome. They also produce more antibodies in response to immunizations.

Studies also consistently show that children who were breastfed as infants suffer less from allergies, asthma, diabetes, colitis, and rheumatoid arthritis. They also have higher I.Q. scores. Breast milk contains special substances that help guide the development of the brain after birth.

Breast milk also safeguards against obesity and cancer. Several carefully designed studies have found that artificially fed infants go on to suffer significantly higher rates of Hodgkin's lymphoma than babies breastfed for six months or more.

And breastfeeding protects your own health. You will bleed less after childbirth. And because breastfeeding suppresses menstruation, you will lose less blood during the chaotic days of early motherhood. You will be at lower risk for hip fracture after menopause. Nursing mothers also have lower rates of ovarian and breast cancer.

And there are practical benefits, too. Breastfeeding can be done one-handed. (Indeed, I'm nursing my son as I'm writing these words.) Bottle-feeding, which takes two hands, makes multi-tasking impossible. Breast milk is so digestible that comparatively little comes out the other end. Less poop. And it has no offensive odor. Really.

On the other hand, the chemical contamination of breast milk is not a trivial issue. When it comes to persistent organic pollutants, breast milk is the most contaminated of all human foods. It typically carries concentrations of organochlorine pollutants that are ten to twenty times higher than those in cow's milk. And children who were breastfed as babies have higher levels of chemical contaminants in their bodies than those who were formula-fed. (Remember, in spite of this fact, breastfed children are healthier, less prone to cancer, and smarter.)

Breast milk is particularly vulnerable to chemical contamination because it exists one rung higher on the human food chain than the food that we adults eat. For chemicals that magnify as they move up the food chain—and the most serious toxins do—our breasts offer the poisons one more chance to concentrate.

DDT and PCBs remain the most widespread contaminants in human milk around the world. Other common contaminants of mother's milk include flame retardants, pesticides, wood preservatives, toilet deodorizers, and dry-cleaning fluids.

BREASTFEEDING RESOURCES

We think every breastfeeding mom should have a copy of *The Nursing Mother's Companion* by Kathleen Huggins. For added encouragement, surf over to:

www.drjacknewman.com
www.lalecheleague.org
www.gotmom.org
www.kellymom.com
www.ilca.org (International Lactation Consultant Association)

drugs and breast milk

Dr. Thomas W. Hale, R.Ph., Ph.D., is a professor of pediatrics at Texas Tech University and a clinical pharmacologist. His four breastfeeding reference books—*Medications and Mothers' Milk, Clinical Therapy in Breastfeeding Patients, Drug Therapy and Breastfeeding: From Theory to Clinical Practice,* and *A Medication Guide for Breastfeeding Moms*—are used throughout the world by physicians, nurses, neonatal NICUs, obstetrical units, and lactation consultants. If you're curious about the effects of a drug you're taking (or thinking of taking) on your breast milk, go to *http://neonatal.ttuhsc.edu/lact.*

Chest Pains: What No One Tells You About Breastfeeding

BY KATE PORTERFIELD

Being pregnant and having a baby is a constant process of having your fantasy of how things are going to be supplanted by the reality of how they are. Nowhere was this more dramatic for me than in the experience of breastfeeding. Before being pregnant, I didn't really know much about nursing, but I certainly had idealized images of it—pictures of nuzzling my baby in the night in a barely lit nursery while my husband slumbered peacefully in the next room. (I would always be seated in an ornate rocking chair, wearing a somewhat Victorian high-necked nightgown in these fantasies—hilarious to consider now when I think about what I was really wearing—usually a stained undershirt that could have used a good wash.) Anyway, my fantasies about breastfeeding were really powerful for me—I simply knew that I had to do this magical thing.

When my first kid was born, having already had the fantasy of childbirth shattered by my actual experience (fantasy: the perfect pushing/breathing/husband-adoring bonding experience; reality: emergency C-section with horrified husband at my head, wincing at the sight of my intestines on the table), I was quick to discover another awful reality: Nursing is unbelievably hard. I literally thought the kid was supposed to just naturally latch on and start sucking. Then, I, in my instinctive, maternal way, would relax and let her eat, organically knowing when to switch to the other side. I seriously thought it would just happen the right way. That is so far from the truth.

Here's what actually happened: my kid latched on in the hospital very shortly after birth. I was psyched. I felt no pain because of post-C-section drugs and I thought we were doing great. By the time I was ready to leave the hospital, I was complaining of a bit of a "twinge" when she latched on. My nipples were getting kind of red and one even had a little cut on it. The nurses were useless. Some recommended Lansinoh (lame—because I was too far beyond for it to help) and some whispered, "I bottle-fed all *my* kids, honey, and they're fine." I left the hospital, still pretty unclear about how it would all work, but pretty sure my kid and I would just get into a rhythm. (This is kind of like thinking you can get married to someone you've known for twenty-five minutes and it'll all "work out.")

When we got home, it got ugly. Things deteriorated on the nipple front really badly—my daughter would suck and suck and I would have no idea whether anything was coming out or not. Sometimes I would let her nurse for like thirty-five minutes on a side. Let me say it again—I had no idea what I was doing. The pain started to be intense when she would latch on. I mean really intense. I mean toes curling, crying, swearing intense. I'm telling you, I was really starting to lose it. I would have to have my mother, husband, or best friend squeeze my toe as hard as they could when she latched on so that I could concentrate on *that* pain rather than the pain of my nipples. Then, I would yell at the person really loudly "Let go!" and tell them they had done it wrong—"God! Can't you just squeeze it when I *tell* you!?" I imagine this would have been really funny to someone watching from outside, but to me, it was just horrible and seemed unable to get any worse.

So, of course, things got worse. Not only did I find myself in total nipple-destruction land, we also discovered at our daughter's one-week pediatric visit that she was losing weight. Badly. What this meant was that, in spite of all the time I was nursing her, she was not getting enough nourishment. My milk had not come in enough and my daughter was also not accessing it well. This was, in hindsight, a good development, because at that point, my doctor said that I needed to go to a lactation consultant if I wanted to keep nursing her. This was a critical moment and I can't quite explain it, but I knew that there was no way I was going to stop nursing her. I truly believed that the only way to feed this child was going to be through my boobs, so, by sending me to a lactation consultant, my doctor was getting me to the person who was going to make that happen.

The details are a bit fuzzy at this point four years later, but the woman was a god-send. She told me that my nipples were the most damaged she had ever seen (an incredibly gratifying piece of news to a semi-psychotic woman who could not stop staring at the—sorry–gaping rivulets of blood that had formed on each nipple) and that my daughter's suck was a "C–." This, too, was gratifying—it was the little punk's fault as much as mine!

What followed was a stringent program that completely consumed me for the next three to four weeks. It involved the following:

- Nipple soaks of warm salt water in a shot glass followed by application of olive oil and, ultimately, bacitracin before and after each feeding
- Pumping as much as possible between feedings to stimulate milk production

- Training my daughter to suck properly using light strokes to her cheeks and tongue (a quite dear process actually)
- Finger-feeding her pumped breast milk with a tiny tube attached to my husband's or mother's pinky finger to give my nipples—and me—a rest. (Why no bottle, you ask? Because, that's how you lose the little devils! Once they get the bottle with its fast flow, they don't want Mama's slow boobs.)
- Daily weigh-ins on a microgram scale to chart our progress
- Nursing as much as was humanly possible, of course

This process was incredible—it started to work within the first few days. My nipples got slightly better and she gained a little bit of weight. This tiny progress was enough for me. It made me absolutely sure that we could succeed. As the weeks passed, my little girl became an A+ sucker and I became adept at feeding her in ways that helped her grow and thrive. It was the happiest experience of my life and the greatest single thing I've ever done. (Until I did it again with number two!)

I honestly don't know how I could have done it without the lactation consultant's involvement. (My husband's constant, unflagging support, by the way, was essential, too.) Almost nothing that she had me do was "instinctual." There is an art and a science to breastfeeding and I had been arrogant to think it was no big deal. Yet I had in me some core belief that if this is what women have been doing for centuries to feed children, then it must be the right way and it must just *happen*. That was my mistake. Something being natural and good for you is not the same as it being easy. So as fantasy world gave way to reality, I discovered that the latter—with all its tears, blood, and toe-squeezing—was a much more gratifying and memorable first experience to have with my daughter. It ain't a Victorian postcard, but it sure was beautiful.

KATE PORTERFIELD is a clinical psychologist and the clinical codirector of the Bellevue/NYU Program for Survivors of Torture at Bellevue Hospital.

postdelivery essentials

Here are a few thoughts on what you'll want to have on hand for postdelivery:

- Maxi pads (unbleached or natural cotton is preferable) in multiple sizes. You may be bleeding for up to six weeks. For pain, a few of these soaked in organic witch hazel, then frozen, can be quite soothing.
- Fragrance-free baby wipes for you. Sometimes toilet paper feels too harsh.
- Hemorrhoid pads, preferably ones containing witch hazel.
- Stool softeners or a lot of dried fruit. You don't want to be straining, especially if you've torn or had an episiotomy.
- Nursing bras. These should be bought a few weeks prior to delivery, at a specialty shop where they can measure you and tell you what you'll need. All-cotton is best. Organic or green cotton is even better. Do not buy anything with an underwire, because it can interfere with milk flow. Your breasts will fluctuate in size as your milk production changes, so don't buy too many at once either.
- If you're modest, you might want to consider nursing tank tops, which will allow you to nurse in public without exposing much more than your nipples. The ones at *www.glamourmom.com* are made from green cotton.
- Sitz bath herbs.
- Cabbage—applying a clean, chilled green leaf can help with breast engorgement, and the leaves are more comfortable than ice packs.

postnatal vitamins

There isn't a huge difference between prenatal and one-a-day vitamins, so after you give birth, you should finish taking your prenatals until you run out, then switch to a regular multivitamin. After you deliver, a nurse will take your blood count. Ask your doctor to let you know if you're deficient in anything and find out exactly how much of any given supplement you'll need daily (iron and calcium are the most common). If you lost a lot of blood, you could be anemic. Strict vegetarians also need to make sure they're getting their daily requirements. Some women find iron supplements constipating and prefer to make up for what they're lacking through diet instead.

If you're exclusively breastfeeding and have a baby born in the Northeast during the winter months, your doctor may suggest giving her vitamin D. (Formula is fortified.) Needless to say, this is controversial. The theory behind this is that winter babies aren't getting enough sunlight, the best source of vitamin D. Food sources aren't very high in D and it only occurs in small amounts in breast milk. The American Academy of Pediatrics recommends drops for all babies because of a rise in rickets (partially due to sunscreens and pollution blocking the sun's rays). Lactation consultants aren't eager to tell parents not to supplement, but they believe breast is best, so it's easy to extrapolate that they don't feel vitamins are necessary. Ultimately it's your choice.

vaccines

Standard protocol for pediatricians is to start administering vaccines for diseases including diphtheria, tetanus, hepatitis B, polio, and pertussis when a baby is two months old. There are parents who try to avoid having these vaccines because they believe they make their children sicker, but the community at large frowns on this. Schools won't accept unvaccinated children, and most pediatricians won't treat unvaccinated babies (or even allow them in their waiting rooms). In response to these strict rules, there are parents who try to space their babies' vaccinations, that is, to have them administered when they're a bit older. This is obviously a personal choice. But it's also a public health concern.

CHAPTER SIXTEEN

fitness

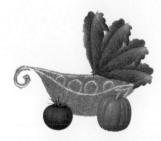

With a new baby, working out may be the last thing on your mind. Or maybe you're dying to go for a run, do an upward facing dog or a back bend, or do all of the other things you've been avoiding in the later stages of your pregnancy. Either way, get your blood moving around your system, even if you're exhausted (if? ha!). It will make you feel better. Most governing bodies (like the American Council on Exercise) tell you to hold off doing anything until six weeks postdelivery, when you get the go-ahead from your doctor.

exercise prior to six weeks

There are little things you can do at home before the doctor's all-clear date. Your activity level pre- and post- that week 6 appointment will have a lot to do with what sort of birth you had. C-section and very torn/episiotomied mommies are less likely to want to hit the treadmill anytime soon. Little extras you can do during the first six weeks include pelvic tilts and deep breathing—filling that somewhat deflated belly up and drawing your navel to your spine when you exhale. Pointing and flexing your feet and moving your legs around can also be done in the early days. But, again, this all depends on how you feel. If you have any pain, pulling, or excessive bleeding, please don't do anything.

goal setting

You probably want to get back to your workout but feel like you don't have the time. Don't set your goals unrealistically high. You might not have an hour to go to the gym. But you could most likely spare ten minutes or so to do sit-ups or modified push-ups or to stretch out. It's hard to get back to working out when you haven't in a while. These little ten-minute bursts will make it easier to get to a gym or a class or outside when and if you have more time. This is not a narcissistic endeavor; it's not just about how you look. Working out can help you with your self-esteem and make you feel strong again.

walking

Walking gets your blood flowing, air into your lungs, and you out of your house. Jogging probably isn't quite in reach yet, as you might leak both urine and breast milk (oh, the joys of motherhood!). Once you're outside, there is no end to what you can organically figure out to do on a park bench. (Speaking of boob leakage, you may need to wear two sports bras during this period, preferably cotton.) Step-ups, squats, stretches, seated ab work—the possibilities are endless. Or just sit there, enjoy the fresh air, and stare at your baby. If you're craving adult companionship, look into some mommy-and-baby group fitness classes.

don't forget to eat

Working out makes you thirsty. Breastfeeding makes you thirsty. So double up on the water. Don't forget to eat, either. Some new moms are so busy, they do just that. Then they work out and get light-headed. Keep snacks in your gym bag, just as you did when you were trying to stave off nausea and just as you will in all bags as soon as your child is old enough to eat solid food.

your aching back

Slings, Björns, breastfeeding, and constantly bending over to lift your baby can put extra strain on your back. When you have time to strengthen your back muscles, go for it. Meanwhile we have a very easy exercise to recommend: think about your posture. Seriously. It's surprising how many times you'll find that you're standing off center. Or maybe you carry your baby on only one hip, throwing your gait all out of whack. This can cause aches and pains everywhere. Channel your inner ballerina. Sit properly (not slumped over) when breastfeeding. If you have a baby carrier that can go on either side of you, wear it on the left side one day and the right side the next. Use your abdominals when walking. Lift the baby, diaper bag, and stroller with your leg and butt muscles; they're much stronger than your lower back. And bend to lift. When pushing a stroller, try not to strangle the grips; this could lead to wrist and forearm pain. Don't push only from your arms, use your legs. Check out your feet. Are you turning your feet out as you walk with a stroller to avoid kicking the wheels? Don't. Have your partner do a fair share of baby-wearing and stroller-pushing, too.

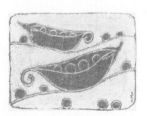

play

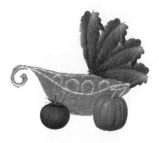

Now for the fun part. Playing with your newborn may feel a little one-sided for the first few months, but that's okay with you. Here are some ideas for the few moments when she isn't eating, sleeping, or having her diaper changed. If you want to get out of the house, it's never too early for the farmers' market.

road trip?

It may seem counterintuitive to have a baby and hit the road a few weeks later as you don't have a care in the world, but we've heard it can actually work surprisingly well. Your newborn spends so much time sleeping and eating that if you weren't so worried about *keeping her from dying*, you'd realize this is a pretty good time to relax. She's portable. Also, you get only one chance to do this, because once number two comes along, it's too late. So plug your rice cooker into the car lighter, pack a cooler, and hit the highway.

infant massage

Baby massage has its roots in India, is regularly practiced in China and throughout Europe, and is growing in popularity in the United States. It's a series of strokes said to calm babies, improve digestion, and offer relief from constipation, colic, and congestion. Some massage-happy parents report they can locate gas bubbles in an upset stomach, and manually rub them out. Studies done at the Touch Research Institute at the University of Miami School of Medicine show premature infants gain more weight when regularly massaged. Many hospitals now offer infant massage classes along with baby care classes. And chic urban mommies are getting in on the trend, too, giving each other private infant-massage-class gift certificates at baby showers. One organic note: Infant massage is best performed with ingestible oils, which can safely be eaten by toe-sucking babies. For more on the subject, check out the bible of baby massage, Vimala McClure's *Infant Massage: A Handbook for Loving Parents.*

Hippie-crite

BY CATHERINE NEWMAN

When I was about a month away from giving birth to my son, a woman in my prenatal yoga class snapped. We were "checking in" like we did, sitting in a circle in some approximation of the lotus position, or what the lotus position might look like as performed by a ring of Humpty Dumpty parade floats. This was Santa Cruz, California, so there was much patchouli in the air, much oneness with nature, much consternation over epidurals and episiotomies. We'd all read *Spiritual Midwifery* and secretly wished that we, too, were giving birth inside a school bus on The Farm in the 1970s, stoned and maybe even stopping to give our husbands a blow job while the "rushes" washed over us. Well, maybe we didn't all wish this. Our teacher had just concluded a fond reminiscence about her own first birthing experience—a vegetable garden featured prominently in the story—when the woman sitting next to me burst into tears. "Look, I'm happy for you that you squatted down in your radish patch and the baby slipped out, okay? But I'm getting an epidural. In fact, if I could, I'd get one now." And then she got galumphingly to her feet, slipped on her Birkenstocks, and left the circle.

We shook our heads pityingly. Poor dupe of The Medical Establishment! And yet I knew that I was more like her than I could say. Not that I didn't want a natural birth—I did. I wanted to labor by the ocean and watch the silvery moonlit waves crash and recede. I wanted a heart brimming with only love as the baby passed easily through me into the world. But I laugh, now, to remember the itemized medical bill that arrived after what was ultimately an abrupted placenta followed by an emergency C-section: the dozens of plastic tubes and surgical dressings and Q-tips and shots of morphine, all mapped out in the cold economy of dollars and cents. Really, my birth was about as natural as Cool Ranch Doritos—and, with the babe swaddled safely in my arms, I was shocked to find that I didn't really care all that much.

But, oh, the pressure to be groovy! I felt it when I was pregnant, and I felt it again, even more acutely perhaps, after the baby was born. Because here's the thing: I don't know what it was like to live on a commune in the seventies—maybe everybody truly did feel as flowy and laid-back as they look in all those naked black-and-white photographs (although I can't help imagining that at least one or two women fantasized about clean sheets or a clean-shaven husband). But to try to live naturally now feels, often, like a contradiction in terms. Like you're part of the very same groovy community that is most anxious about the dangers of the world and the precariousness of your baby's well-being. And so I am, at my very grooviest, simultaneously most neurotic—like some kind of a hippie catch-22. As a spank-ing-new mother, I strolled through the farmers' market with my baby asnooze in an organic cotton sling, chatting with the growers about Gaia melons and Jewel yams—while my mind raced with worries. Circumcision. Vaccinations. Fluoride. Pesticides. Toxins in breast milk. Mercury. The baby was so beautiful, and yet I fretted myself into a knot.

And maybe that's what it has to be like—maybe you have to learn to live with contra-dictions. To be the earth-goddess-mama you want to be, maybe you have to suffer through a certain amount of neurosis. If you're like me, then maybe you can hate TV and rail against The System, defend the family bed, and spackle mashed organic bananas into your baby's mouth—but also believe that antibiotics and a C-section saved your life. Maybe while you're breastfeeding, you're wishing you had a Diet Coke. Maybe after you got home from the hospital, you chewed and swallowed dozens of miniature candy bars left over from Halloween—just your everyday Almond Joy and Bit-O-Honey, nothing sustainably grown or dotted with spelt husks—even though the gulp-gulping of the baby from the spigots of your body made real your connection in a way that the abstracted amniotic osmosing never quite could. Maybe your baby got a rash from cloth diapers, so you switched, sheepishly, to disposables. Maybe you bought a "conventional" lemon at the Whole Foods Market because you just couldn't shell out the cash for organic citrus— but maybe you bought it furtively, stashing it beneath your kale (along with the organic coffee and spirulina-fed pork) like you were shoplifting. Maybe you felt specious, wielding British breastfeeding lore about the benefits of lager, when all you really wanted was to justify cracking open a beer once the baby was asleep. Maybe for an entire week you ate barbequed chicken legs from a two-gallon Ziploc bag because a friend brought them over and they were on the top shelf of the fridge and, with the baby in the Björn, you couldn't bend down to reach the apples in the produce drawer. And also you were just so tired.

I don't mean to be glib. It's an immoderate world, and so we must take immoderate measures to safeguard the health of ourselves and our children. I'm just saying roll with it a little. Don't worry more than you need to—or weigh yourself down with the burden of guilt. Because chances are there's weight enough, what with that little milk-fed pumpkin dangling from your neck in a sling. And maybe you'll never feel quite right—not in front of your father, who looks away whenever you feed the baby, as if perhaps your entire body has been appliquéd with breasts and World's Most Grotesque Hippie is tattooed on your forehead, and not in front of your earthier-than-thou mama friend, who doesn't even laugh politely when you joke, "Maybe I should just put it directly into his bottle," before swigging from your margarita while the baby nurses. But, not to get all Mr. Rogers on you, I think you're okay just the way you are. I think you're probably doing your best. And when you rock that little baby in the hush of the night, when you stroke the curve of his cheek in the moonlight, when you lean in to inhale his milky, perfect breath—well, you'll probably think that doing your best is actually as good as it gets.

CATHERINE NEWMAN *writes "Bringing Up Ben & Birdy," an online column at* www.babycentre.com, *and is the author of the memoir* Waiting for Birdy.

generation gap

Until now you've had total control over what you feed your baby, but soon other people will be involved in the process, so it's important to stick to your guns without seeming unappreciative. This is a great place to get your partner involved, especially if his or her parents are going to be babysitting and aren't that enthused about organic food, glass bottles, and wooden toys. You might be feeling less than justified making demands and requests, but you've invested an awful lot of energy to not follow through now. If you're visiting relatives or friends, just fill up your car with your own groceries before you arrive. You'll be happy to have what you need, and they'll be happy because they don't have to worry about you. When it comes time to feed the baby solid food and someone's babysitting at your house, just let them know that you have all the food the baby will need. The point is to be firm, but not make a huge fuss. There's not a single person with a kid who doesn't impose on somebody, so don't feel like you have to apologize for yours.

the ten-minute "mobile"

The going thought is that contrasting black-and-white images enthrall and stimulate newborns. Most store-bought mobiles contain black-and-white swirly tops, along with the bells, whistles, and lights that entertain babies. If you're not interested in dropping fifty bucks on a plastic mobile that may or may not turn your baby into Einstein, but that she certainly won't get much use out of beyond month 5, make your own. You do too have time. At 4 A.M. when your husband is rocking her back to sleep and you're on standby, ready to nurse in case it doesn't work. Grab a black marker and some white paper. Draw circles, big stripes, checkerboards, and swirls, then tack them to surfaces your baby stares at most often—on the wall to the side of the changing table, above your bed, on the walls near her bed, above the kitchen sink where you bathe her. Besides cost, and keeping another plastic toy out of a landfill, who knows? Maybe it will turn her into a genius after all.

The Organic Crowd

BY JACK HITT

The first time I ever gave the word *organic* a moment's thought was after my daughters were born. The urban legend at the time was that store-bought hormone-saturated industrial-bred cow's milk would cause both infant daughters to develop breasts when they were nine years old. I had seen a neighborhood girl hit puberty at that age. Unable to understand what was happening, she suddenly looked out at the world with eyes full of terror, as if an alien being had invaded her body and might at any minute begin rippling wildly beneath her skin.

So, I bought the organic milk. It came in a carton as blue as a spring sky with a cartoon cow ruminating in a meadow on the front. I liked seeing its cozy image when I opened the icebox, and I preferred to see it at the houses of other parents with infant children, too. Then a friend of mine who grew his own organic food and studied these issues deeply told me that in the part of New England where I live, the dairy cows are not primed with growth hormone, so regular milk sold in the milky-colored plastic jugs for $1.75 a half gallon is about as organic as my pastoral brand, sold for three bucks.

I resisted this information at first. And then I started wondering why I was resisting this information (which is why I can be an infuriating writer but a decent husband). Could it be that I had been seduced by carton design? Or was it that I wanted other people to see my blue carton and know that I was the kind of parent who understands the ramifications of modern food, especially for growing girls, and took action? Maybe it was just that buying something clearly designated organic relieved my wife and me, and us alone, of the stress that comes with worrying about our kids' welfare.

Still, I couldn't resist the facts as I had learned them. The cheaper milk might signify something different, but it was essentially the same thing. Being a cheapskate at heart, I started buying regular milk. When other parents came over and I saw them seeing me pour what they considered poison into their child's bottle, I would find myself unable to resist telling them the "facts." This is one of the joys and annoyances of knowing a smarty-pants journalist. We're constantly telling you all about what you don't know. As I've discovered so many times, facts don't really count for much, and they're no match for the weighty unconscious assumptions that undergird a word like *organic*. My facts and I were able to convert a total of zero parents to the view that the cheaper, mass-produced dull-white-container milk was just as good as the premium, small-farm variety with its *Goodnight Moon* cover design.

So, having resisted the facts before wondering about them, I was now wondering why my wondering had not caused anyone else to wonder (which is why I can also be an infuriating husband but a decent writer). The word *organic* is one of those verbal oddities in American English, a kind of linguistic sponge. While it might have a very specific, regulation-specific, Department of Agriculture dictionary meaning, it also drags a long chain of connotations in its wake.

In pop culture, too, the word has taken on all kinds of associations—most curiously, religious ones. By religion, I don't mean the kind of religion I grew up with—the going-to-church religion. That was religion that existed in the present tense. We went to church (which was boring), but afterward we'd check in with people gathered in the parish hall for coffee and for something much bigger. My childhood congregation at St. Philips in Charleston, South Carolina, is 300 years old, and the sense of tradition that ruled over that coffee hour provided a solid feeling about the larger world beyond. Yet, as a kid, what I loved about church was that coffee hour—that time when a hundred or so like-minded people showed up once a week to break a little bread and feel the connectedness of a community that's come together, traditionally.

But that's not the religious I'm talking about. Organic seems to fire up the apocalyptic in us—religion in the future tense. Americans love to see things in these terms. It's been a pretty common reaction ever since the Puritans first looked into the misty colonial woods of America's seventeenth century and saw flying devils.

For instance, the widow of Grateful Dead guitarist Jerry Garcia is a filmmaker named Deborah Koons Garcia. She made a popular film called *The Future of Food*. It's shown regularly at house parties where the message is preached to larger audiences. Garcia takes the acknowledged facts about modern food—that it's been mechanized and industrialized and capitalized—and sees a coming apocalypse.

"Someone needed to make this film, because if this technology isn't challenged and if this corporatization of our whole food system isn't stopped, at some point it will be too late," she told *Wired* magazine. By "too late," she meant that we would all be poisoned by the new food demons that swoop around us like the forest fiends that harassed the original pilgrims: Frankenfoods. Irradiation. "Mad Cow" disease. Bovine growth hormone. Genetically modified plants. Toxic sludge fertilizer. Cloned animals.

Organic for some folks is not just a word; it is a revelation. Forget the hormone or pesticide regulations—organic can signify a choice between good and evil. This sentiment has taken hold, and it's why even companies like Wal-Mart are willing to fly in their organic food from halfway around the word to sell its branded wholesomeness at its stores. Is a rasher of bacon from a pig raised on locals' acorns, but then flown in from several continents away at an expense of tanks of jet fuel, still "organic"? There might be an argument there, but not to the maestros of modern grocery-store economics. There, the acorn-fed pig is all good, and hogs in North Carolina dwelling beside sweltering lagoons of urine and consuming industrial slop are bad.

Around the time that I gave up on the sky-blue organic milk for the heretical reasoning that the facts didn't support the higher cost, I started shopping at my local farmers' market. I live in Connecticut, which is a strange little state. It's known as a rich bedroom community for wealthy Wall Street tycoons who hate the idea of living in Manhattan. But in fact the state is a wild mix of micro-communities—ethnic outposts, corrupt urban harbor towns, villages of rednecks (who look very familiar to a Southerner like me), and, more inland, a rural and agricultural stretch. Each spring, this last set fans out to the various cities on the weekend and sells its produce.

The reason I started shopping at the farmers' market was quite capitalistic. I liked the freshness of all that I bought. Plus, farmers who cater to these new outposts—there are now farmers' markets in nearly every town in Connecticut—are exquisitely attuned to our demands.

Shoppers at farmers' markets tend to be people who've figured out not only that the food in grocery stores is not, by any definition, organic, but also that these little farmers' markets offer a variety that is devastating when compared to the big box supermarkets. New things appear every week. All sorts of melons and greens and other items simply too delicate for the brutal shipping and shelf demands of a supermarket are commonplace. The food follows the seasonal harvests. Much of the conversation is about getting to know the food, how it's grown and how to prepare it. "Organic" is at the heart of these markets, and as a result, the food feels more real.

The thing about grocery stores is that they are mostly illusion. Variety appears to be all over the place because Super Stop & Shops are architectural cocoons of psychedelic color and brisk Muzak. But the truth is that while the fruits and vegetables section might boast a few star fruits or pomelos, the big bins are packed with the same old Florida oranges, Idaho potatoes, and Washington apples that they know sell in the mass market.

There was a scandal here a while back that beautifully captured the nuances of modern choice at the grocery store. One of the owners was busted for selling fake mesclun, the delicacy composed of baby lettuces of many varieties. Cooks love it because mesclun tends to be a mix of tastes, including some sharply bitter arugula. It's also colorful, filled with crimsons and pastel greens and browns and whites. Radicchio with its purples and snowy outer edges give any pack of mesclun a cool, sophisticated look.

It's also very expensive. Mesclun can run up to $10 a pound. That's way more than iceberg lettuce, the middlebrow green that has fed America since World War II, that can cost as little as a few dimes a pound. So the scandal was this: The grocery store owner was taking older iceberg that was going bad and cutting it up into little pieces. He'd throw in a piece or two of radicchio to give it color, plus some small spinach leaves, and then sell it as mesclun. Suddenly, something that once fetched 39 cents a pound was $10 a pound. Nice work if you can get it.

But that's not the real scandal. After the fake mesclun was exposed, one of the store owners was quoted as saying that the real reason he did it was because the fake mesclun *outsold* the authentic stuff. It was hard to read that story and not come away thinking that while Americans proclaim their love of choice and fresh flavors, what many *really* want is what they've always known. This grocer had just figured out the paradox behind a lot of American shopping: We want to buy the *idea* of exotic food and unusual tastes, but take home the reality of comfort food and familiar flavors. And we get exactly what we want for the low, low price of $10 a pound. Who can really blame the grocer?

Around this time, I first came across another variation of the word *organic*. Religious fundamentalists use the word. They refer disparagingly to something called "organic evolution." It's meant to signify the heathen belief that evolution happens without the guiding hand of God—that is, organically. The folks fighting food corruption share with the biblical literalists a certain understanding. Both believe the word involves some aspect of man's arrogance. The fundamentalists see human pride in the idea that mere science adequately explains the magnificence of Nature, and the foodies see man's arrogance in the reckless faith that we can interfere in the food chain without catastrophic results. Both uses of the word summon a sense that a great moral choice is being made.

I find myself backing away from the word when I get that sense that a large moral mandate is being forced upon me. My maverick self eagerly learns the facts and buys the cheap milk. Still, I find myself veering toward goods sold as organic. I want my food to be pure, or at least fussed over. So, I go to the farmers' market, not because the world's coming to an end, but maybe because a new one's beginning. The farmers' market happens near a public square on the other side of town. My little girls and I make a point of going almost every Saturday. We've gotten to know the cranky guy who sells the heirloom tomatoes, the young father who grass-feeds his own cows in Old Lyme, and the migrant workers who always show up with the yellowest wax beans and the rosiest pears and the greenest rabe. There's also the Yale students who grow all kinds of stuff I've never heard of in some greenhouses near the Divinity School. They accompany every sale with a long and energetic story about how each vegetable is grown. I suspect they might find the word *organic* too frivolous a term to capture the high-minded environmental science that goes into the nurturing of their tasty, misshapen yellow beets.

The whole thing happens under a bunch of tents. People mingle for about an hour. Coffee gets served, and sometimes the bread folks have some great treats for both kids and adults. We hang out for a while, and the girls see old friends they used to know from swimming lessons or the old preschool crowd they grew up with or that music class they abandoned a long time ago.

I don't know how orthodoxed organic it really is. The cow guy once confessed that he bought his calves from a feed lot where they ate corn. With some of the vegetable people you get a hesitant grin and a lot of tangled sentences if you ask about pesticides. I can't speak for the food, technically. But I can speak for the people. We like them, and we trust them. On some level, it's the opposite of the grocery store. I have no idea where the food there came from and would never be bothered to learn. But here at the market the food comes directly from these people we know. Every spring, my family comes out of the cold, reconvenes with this old crowd, and we buy our local food. My girls like to check in with these people we see only occasionally. On some level, it's nothing more than just a hundred or so like-minded people who show up once a week to break a little bread and feel the connectedness of a community that's come together, organically.

JACK HITT is a contributing writer for the New York Times Magazine, Harper's Magazine, *and the public radio program* This American Life.

beauty

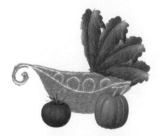

You made it. Like so much in your life now, this section has more to do with your baby than you. Don't worry; we have tips for you, too. Now for the good stuff.

chapped nipples

These are a fact of breastfeeding life, especially when you're getting started. Kirstin Binder at SaffronRouge suggests Primavera's rose floral water; Kate Sharp, a New York–based lactation consultant, prefers warm soaks with a washcloth or saltwater soaks a few times a day. Make a saltwater solution—about a teaspoon of salt in a cup of water—and wet your nipples with it. Many women find these soaks work as well as nipple creams (which don't allow for air circulation). Olive oil can also provide relief and is safe for a baby to swallow. If you don't like the feeling of plain oil on your nipples, try Motherlove nipple cream (olive oil is the main ingredient). Always read labels for base oils and for the fewest amount of ingredients possible. Vitamin E isn't safe for infants to eat and often comes in a wheat germ oil base. Wheat is a potential allergen. We recognize that these are your nipples we're talking about. How you deal with them is your business. Really bad chapping and cracking can make you want not to breastfeed. If you can't get the relief you want with the remedies suggested above, there's always

Lansinoh. It's basically purified lanolin. No word on if the sheep are organic, but as conventional remedies go, it has the market cornered. It also scores well in terms of safety concerns in the Environmental Working Group's Skin Deep report, and La Leche promotes it, so it can't be too bad.

stretch marks

Stretch marks don't go away just because your belly deflates (or starts to). For some people, blackthorn oil (Dr. Hauschka makes one) can help heal this fact of life. So can some of the belly oils you may have been using prior to giving birth. Slather it on. And remember, stretch marks fade with time, too.

hair dye, nail polish, and everything else you gave up for the last nine months

You've already cleaned up your act and probably even found some good new products, so why return to your old, chemical ways? Especially when breastfeeding. If there is something you're just dying to do, check with a lactation consultant or doctor. Also before you go spraying your favorite pre-pregnancy perfume all over yourself, think of all the time you spend nuzzling your baby's whisper-thin skin. You should try to be just as fragrance-free as the laundry detergent and baby wipes you buy to keep the baby rash-free.

bathing baby

As with everything baby, there are schools of thought about how to bathe your child from the minute she's born. It's almost impossible to get your baby home from a hospital unbathed. The midwivery community thinks you shouldn't bathe a baby just after birth because the scent of amniotic fluid on her hands makes her more interested in nursing. They also feel if there is any vernix left on the baby (the creamy, white substance that coats and protects the baby's skin in utero), it should be left where it is because it's great for her skin. There's also a concern that a bath right after birth will make a baby too cold. Hospitals usually place newborns in warmers until their temperature rises again, forcing the baby and mom to miss out on early bonding hours. Once home, parents are advised to just sponge bathe their children until the umbilical cord falls off. After this happens, some parents start using a plastic baby tub. Others "family bathe"—where one parent gets in the tub with the baby and washes her, then hands her off to the dry parent. Never get in and out of a tub holding a wet baby because both are very slippery. Whatever you decide to do, remember babies don't get that dirty. You need to concentrate on only a few areas—their neck folds (which collect breast milk and formula) and the creases of their thighs. Don't forget behind the ears and in between their little fingers and toes. Mild baby soaps are good for bodies and hair (Weleda's calendula products for babies are universally loved). In general, avoid all creams, shampoos, and ointments unless really needed.

powder

Even though most powder is referred to as baby powder, don't use any on your baby. Not only do some powders contain talc, which is a carcinogen, but powder can irritate babies' airways when inhaled. People think powder is absorbent, but it can actually increase dampness, bacterial growth, and rashes.

organic cotton

Once you start to embrace organic living, you may find yourself thinking about your cotton washcloths, cotton swabs, and cotton balls. Cotton is one of the largest crops grown in America. Luckily all of these are available in organic cotton versions which, like organic lettuce, adhere to regulated government standards. Added bonus: organic cotton doesn't contain chlorine bleach and is less likely to irritate baby skin. This is good news for parents who use cotton squares with water in place of wipes.

baby nails

Baby nails grow very fast and will need to be cut more often than yours. If you're worried about cutting her skin, push the finger pad away as you trim. Try infant nail scissors instead of clippers. Some nail-trimming-impaired parents put gloves or mittens on their babies so they won't scratch their own faces, but a baby mouthing at her hands or trying to suck her knuckles is an early sign of hunger, which comes a few stages before crying. And the gloves can get in the way. You will nick her most likely at some point during pruning. Things happen. You're not a bad parent.

wipes

You'll soon be an expert on diaper changing, but here's a tip for the first few days: bring oil with you to the hospital—olive oil, calendula oil, or something equally mild. The first poop—called meconium—is extremely sticky. If you coat your baby's bottom with oil first, it makes the poop slide right off. The less wiping, the less tears. After that, warm water and washcloths will suffice. If you prefer baby wipes, buy pure, alcohol- and fragrance-free versions. Tushies makes them. So does Seventh Generation.

diaper cream

Your baby will develop a rash at some point. Sensitive skin wrapped tightly in a layer of acidic moisture and poop irritates skin. Most diaper rash creams contain zinc oxide, which acts as both a barrier and an astringent. This targets the fungi that cause the rash. Our diaper cream of choice is made by Weleda. It has a low percentage of zinc oxide mixed with organic ingredients. If your baby is rashy all the time, you can use it preventatively as a barrier, but don't use cream if your baby doesn't need it. The problem with preventative care is that it doesn't allow the skin to breathe. If you have an opportunity, try airing out the baby's tush.

blocking the sun's rays

The general consensus is that kids under six months should not be wearing sun-block, nor should they be in the direct sun. If you live in a sunny climate or have a summer baby, invest in hats, umbrellas, and other coverings. If you're keen on using sunblock before six months, check with your doctor and then use a brand that contains the least amount of chemicals. Most sunblocks contain a fair amount of suspected carcinogens. Zinc oxide and titanium dioxide are said to effectively block the sun while resting on top of the skin instead of getting absorbed into it. It's not always possible to find sunblocks that contain the right ingredients, are organic, and are safe for kids. Organic options include Dr. Hauschka and any made by Lavera (they even have one chlorophyll-dyed green version so you can see where it has and hasn't covered). Other (nonorganic) but pretty pure versions include Burt's Bees, California Baby, and Blue Lizard Baby.

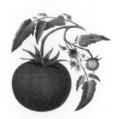

CHAPTER EIGHTEEN

so now what?

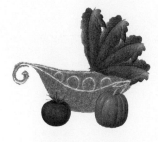

You had the organic pregnancy; you birthed the organic baby. Your diet is ideal for breastfeeding. You're a pro at eating whole foods. The nursery (and your home) is nontoxic down to the paint on the walls, and so are the cleaning products under your kitchen sink. Maybe you even know the characters at your local farmers' market by name. You have glass baby bottles but don't sweat the occasional plastic water bottle. The creams in your bathroom are so pure they're practically edible, and none of them contain anything that would irritate your baby when nuzzling. You're pretty much set. What next?

Maintenance.

Sure, we could walk you through every milestone, showing you the organic way. Sleep deprivation, teething, weaning, babyproofing, playgroups, first steps, first colds, toddler beds, and so on. We think that you having read the previous pages put you in a mind-set to meet new challenges, any challenges, organically. We've given you the tools to do what we do as our babies grow: question everything that surrounds them and goes in or on them—from clothes to water to medicine to toys to day care. You get the point. Be skeptical. Don't just blindly trust your pediatricians or your in-laws. Advice is to be taken with a grain of salt. Research. Try to come up with the best, safest, most organic solutions that will benefit not only our babies but the world they're inheriting. To that end, we want to stress the importance of continuing what you've already started: living a complete organic life.

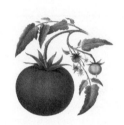

breakfast, lunch, dinner, pickles, ice cream, and baby food

BREAKFAST

MISO SOUP WITH TOFU AND SPINACH

from Nora Pouillon, chef/owner of Nora's and Asia Nora in Washington, D.C., America's first certified organic restaurant

. . . .

"It's easier to get yourself off caffeine by first switching to decaf," Pouillon says. "I substituted coffee with miso soup in the morning, especially in the winter. In all of the Asian cultures, they have a nourishing meal with tofu in the morning—something that gives you energy longer than sugar and coffee. You can put all kinds of vegetables in it or none at all. I think of pregnancy as a way of life, not a disease."

SOUP
4 cups dashi vegetable stock or water
¼ cup red miso paste, or more to taste
6 tablespoons thinly sliced scallions
1 teaspoon minced garlic (optional)
8 shiitakes, sliced
Tofu, cut up into small cubes (optional)
Spinach, julienned (optional)

1 tablespoon rice wine vinegar

2 tablespoons minced fresh ginger, or to taste

1 teaspoon honey or sugar

¼ teaspoon minced jalapeño or ground black pepper

1. Combine the seasoning ingredients, mix well, and set aside at room temperature.
2. In a stainless steel saucepan, bring 2 cups of the vegetable stock to a boil, reduce the heat to a simmer, and whisk in the miso until it is dissolved.
3. Add the scallions and garlic.
4. Add the remaining 2 cups vegetable stock to the miso soup; do not let boil.
5. Simmer for 5 to 10 minutes and then add the shiitakes, and the tofu and spinach, if you are using them.
6. Add the seasoning, about 2 teaspoons per serving. Serve hot.

SERVES 4

LUNCH

ORGANIC HEIRLOOM TOMATO SALAD

from Ben Ford, chef and proprietor of Ford's Filling Station in Culver City, California

"This salad was great for us," says Ford, a father of one who teaches classes at Garden Magic Kids, a nonprofit group dedicated to planting organic gardens in urban public schools. "We had the pleasure of experiencing a summertime pregnancy, and we could prepare this with ingredients from our own garden."

SALAD

1 head frisee lettuce

4 large heirloom tomatoes

1 pound mozzarella cheese (or Burrata, if you can find it and it's pasteurized)

⅓ cup sherry vinaigrette (see below)

1 teaspoon coarse sea salt
1 tablespoon coarse black pepper

SHERRY VINAIGRETTE
2 caramelized shallots
½ cup sherry vinegar
2 tablespoons late harvest Reisling vinegar
1½ cups extra-virgin olive oil
1 pinch kosher salt

1. Whisk salt into vinegar to dissolve. Add shallots while whisking slowly. Add olive oil. Season to taste. (This will make more than you need for this salad. Refrigerate and use as desired.)
2. Discard dark portions of frisee.
3. Cut tomatoes in four thick slices.
4. Portion the cheese into four pieces.
5. Lightly toss frisee with sherry vinaigrette, making small nests on the plate.
6. Layer the tomatoes with a small amount of sherry vinaigrette.
7. Gently layer the cheese on the top of stacked tomatoes and sprinkle with a layer of salt.
8. Sprinkle the plate with cracked black pepper.

SERVES 4

WATERMELON SALAD

from Amanda Hesser, food editor of the New York Times Magazine

"The one long feast that I imagined pregnancy would be sadly did not occur. For much of my pregnancy with twins, I was more in touch with my survival instincts than my epicurean side. In the beginning I felt like a sick animal, uninterested in eating, just trying to get through days filled with nausea.

The few cravings I had were alarmingly odd. For the first three months, all I wanted were Fritos, Duchy Originals oaten biscuits, and citrus fruits. Eventually this shifted to oshinko (Japanese pickles) and, toward the end, to watermelon. Once I could muster up the energy, I began to introduce the babies to as many flavors as possible, in the hopes that they would welcome a wide range of foods once they were born. This was based on nothing scientific, just instinct. I ate Korean, Thai, Spanish, French, Jewish deli food, Moroccan, and the like. The only food they thoroughly rejected was Raisin Bran. And who can blame them?"

¼ seedless watermelon
1½ cups halved ripe cherry tomatoes
2 teaspoons slivered mint leaves
2 tablespoons extra-virgin olive oil
Salt
Freshly ground black pepper
½ lemon

Using a melon baller, carve out 2 cups of balls from the watermelon. Reserve the rest of the watermelon for another use. In a large serving bowl, gently blend the watermelon balls with the tomatoes, mint, and olive oil. Season with salt, pepper, and lemon juice.

SERVES 4

MIXED BABY GREENS WITH CURRY VINAIGRETTE

from Myra Goodman, founder of California's Earthbound Farms

"I can't remember a specific salad (my last delivery was thirteen years ago!), but I always ate lots of salads," says Goodman. "Spring mix has so many more vitamins than iceberg, as well as fiber, and sitting down with a huge bowl of salad on my belly and eating it with my fingers was definitely a daily occurrence."

This vinaigrette works especially well with the nuts, seeds, and fruit that adorn this salad.

VINAIGRETTE
2 tablespoons red wine vinegar
½ cup extra-virgin olive oil
1 tablespoon Dijon mustard
1 tablespoon plus 1 teaspoon curry powder
¼ teaspoon salt

SALAD
½ cup whole pecans
⅓ cup pumpkin seeds
8 ounces Earthbound Farms organic mixed baby greens
1 Earthbound Farms organic Fuji or Gala apple, diced
⅓ cup Earthbound Farms organic raisins

1. Combine the vinaigrette ingredients in a jar and shake vigorously to combine.
2. In a skillet, toast the pecans until fragrant, watching carefully to prevent burning. Let cool and then coarsely chop.
3. Toast the pumpkin seeds in the same manner until lightly browned.
4. Place the greens in a large bowl with the pecans, pumpkin seeds, apple, and raisins. Add about half of the dressing and toss thoroughly. Add more vinaigrette if needed. Serve immediately.

SERVES 6 TO 8

SPRING TONIC NETTLE SOUP

from Jessica Prentice, professional chef and cookbook author

. . . .

"Nettles are an excellent food for women at all reproductive stages because they are very rich in iron. Women lose a good deal of iron through menstruation, but also through the placenta during childbirth and through breastfeeding afterward. This soup is a simple and wonderful way to eat fresh nettles, which can be found at farmers' markets or growing wild in the countryside—especially in spring. Do not handle nettles with bare hands, as they sting. Use tongs or a glove. The sting is deactivated with cooking."

(The following recipe is reprinted from *Full Moon Feast: Food and the Hunger for Connection*, by Jessica Prentice. Used by permission of Chelsea Green Publishing, Inc., copyright © 2006.)

2 leeks, cut into rounds
3 tablespoons butter or olive oil
¼ pound stinging nettle tops
1 bay leaf or bouquet garni
1 quart light chicken stock or filtered water
2 egg yolks
½ cup crème fraîche
Salt and pepper to taste
Nutmeg to taste

1. Sauté the leeks in the butter or olive oil.
2. Add the nettles (being careful not to touch them with your bare hands!), bay leaf or bouquet garni, and stock or water.
3. Cover, bring to a boil, and simmer until the nettles are very soft.
4. Meanwhile, in a bowl, whisk together the egg yolks and crème fraîche.
5. Remove the bay leaf or bouquet garni from the soup, turn the heat to low, and purée using an immersion blender, adding a generous pinch of salt and a grind of pepper.
6. Take a ladleful of soup and stir it into the egg mixture.

7. Return the egg-nettle mixture to the soup and stir gently over very low heat (do not let it boil again).
8. Grate some fresh nutmeg into the soup, taste, and add more salt as necessary to make it savory and delicious.

Variation: Add a handful of sorrel leaves to the soup for a lemony flavor.

SERVES 4

DINNER

GREEN RICE WITH ROASTED GREEN CHILIES AND LEEKS

*from Deborah Madison, author of 8 cookbooks and founding chef of
San Francisco's Greens Restaurant*

. . . .

"What are you going to make with all those leeks?' I had to ask Nicole, who was eight months pregnant and standing in the produce section of the market with her arms full of leeks. Most people don't buy leeks by the armfuls, but Nicole's enthusiastic answer—green rice with chilies and leeks!—inspired me to go home and make this dish, and I'm glad I did. It's comfort and joy for those who are soothed by rice that comes with a chili fix—pregnant or not. (Both Nicole and I live in New Mexico, where chilies do bring comfort!) Sometimes I serve this with Mexican oregano, quartered limes, and sliced avocado. But plain is good, too. This is a filling weeknight sort of a dish, to which I might add a colorful vegetable for an appetizer, such as vinegared beets nested in their greens, or a jícama, orange, and avocado salad."

3 cups chicken stock, vegetable stock, or water
6 leeks, the white parts plus the paler greens (about 3 cups chopped)
1 cup fresh parsley leaves
½ cup fresh cilantro leaves
Sea salt
3 poblano chilies or 4 to 5 Anaheim chilies
1 to 2 tablespoons vegetable oil

1½ cups rice (short- or long-grain)
1 bay leaf
1 to 2 ounces jack or Muenster cheese, cubed
½ cup sour cream, loosened and stirred with a fork

1. If you're making the vegetable stock, start it first: Put the leek roots and lighter green leek trimmings in a pot with 5 cups water, a grated carrot, a handful of parsley and cilantro stems, a pinch each of thyme and oregano, and ½ teaspoon salt. Bring to a boil and simmer, uncovered, for 25 minutes. Strain.
2. Char the chilies over a flame, then drop them in a bag to steam for 15 minutes. Slip off the skins, pull out the seeds, and chop into ½-inch pieces.
3. Heat the oil in a Dutch oven. Add the rice and cook, stirring occasionally, over medium-high heat for about 5 minutes. Add the leeks, chilies, bay leaf, 1 teaspoon salt, and the 3 cups stock or water. Give a stir, cook for a few minutes, then lower the heat. Cover and simmer for 20 minutes.
4. While the rice is cooking, purée the parsley and cilantro with 1 cup water or any extra stock. When the rice is done, stir the purée into it and add the cheese. Swirl in the sour cream just before serving for a pretty white-and-green effect.

SERVES 4

CHICKEN SOUP AND ROSEMARY DUMPLINGS

from Dan Barber, chef/co-owner of Blue Hill at Stone Barns in Pocantico Hills, New York

"Chicken soup is comforting to whoever eats it," Barber pronounces. This goes double for pregnant women.

CHICKEN SOUP

4 large onions, cut into small dice
4 carrots, peeled and cut into small dice

2 ribs celery, cut into small dice

5 pounds chicken wings

Sherry vinegar

7 pounds cut-up chicken bodies—feet, etc.

3 onion brûlée

5 bay leaves

2 heads garlic, split

Salt and pepper

Water

5 bunches thyme

2 sprigs rosemary

1. Slowly caramelize the onions in a small rondeau or heavy saucepan.
2. When the onions are well sweated and lightly colored, add the rest of the mirepoix (vegetables) and cook until well caramelized.
3. Split the wings at the joints and in a large rondeau brown the wings to dark golden brown. Remove, do a second batch of wings. Remove.
4. Drain the large rondeau of the fat, deglaze with sherry vinegar, reduce, and add the browned wings, mirepoix, chicken parts, brûlée, bay leaves, garlic, and salt and pepper to taste. Add water to cover all of the ingredients. Bring to a light simmer and keep there for a while. After 3 hours, add the thyme and rosemary.
5. Adjust the seasoning throughout; skim throughout.
6. When good chicken flavor has been achieved, strain through a china cap and then through a chinois.

SERVES 8

ROSEMARY DUMPLINGS

4 eggs, separated

2 cups matzo meal

2 ounces foie gras fat

4 ounces club soda

2 sprigs rosemary, diced to dust

2 scallions, sliced as thin as possible

Salt and pepper

1 quart chicken stock (for cooking dumplings)

1. In an aluminum bowl, using a rubber spatula, combine the egg yolks, matzo, foie gras fat, club soda, rosemary, scallions, and salt and pepper to taste.
2. In a separate aluminum bowl, whip the egg whites to soft peaks.
3. Fold into the batter lightly. The batter should be thin at this point. Bring the chicken stock to a light simmer. When the batter has solidified so that it can be rolled into little balls about the diameter of a nickel or quarter, slowly add them to the poaching liquid, no more than 10 at a time. When quite firm but just slightly raw, remove and place in a warm container with warm stock to cover. Either use or refrigerate.

When serving the soup, include a nice selection of seasonal vegetables, dumplings, chicken breast, and chicken leg.

YIELDS 64 SMALL DUMPLINGS

BUTTERNUT SQUASH ERISHERI

from Maya Kaimal, author of *Curried Favors* and *Savoring the Spice Coast of India,* and founder, Maya Kaimal Fine Indian Foods

"My husband and I launched our Indian sauce company while I was pregnant with twins. While developing the recipes, I stood over countless steam kettles inhaling curry and vindaloo vapors—thankfully never once feeling queasy. It must have seeped into Anna's and Lucy's subconscious, because now (at two) curry and rice is one of their favorite meals.

"This recipe is one that all of us enjoy. It's very nutritious, contains little oil, and has an unexpectedly sweet twist from deeply toasted coconut. It comes from the southwestern Indian state of Kerala, where my father was raised, and where nearly every dish includes some form of coconut. Fresh curry leaves give it an authentic Kerala aroma, but it will be quite delicious without them, especially when made with a rich organic butternut squash. Serve with steamed basmati rice and a favorite chicken curry or green vegetable."

    1 cup grated unsweetened coconut
    1 organic butternut squash
    ¼ teaspoon turmeric
    ¼ teaspoon cayenne
    1¼ teaspoons salt
    ½ teaspoon chopped garlic
    1 teaspoon cumin seeds
    ½ cup canned organic pinto beans
    2 tablespoons vegetable oil
    1 teaspoon mustard seeds
    2 dried red chilies
    1 sprig fresh curry leaves (optional)

1. In a dry frying pan, toast ½ cup of the coconut over medium heat, stirring constantly until it turns the color of cinnamon and no white remains. Be careful not to burn it. Set aside.
2. Peel the squash, halve it lengthwise, and scoop out the seeds. Cut into ¾-inch cubes and measure 4 cups, reserving any extra for another use.
3. In a deep, wide pan, combine the squash, turmeric, cayenne, salt, and 1½ cups water. Bring to a boil, reduce the heat, and simmer, covered, until the squash is tender and begins to break down when stirred (20 to 25 minutes).
4. While the squash is cooking, combine in a blender the remaining ½ cup coconut, the garlic, and the cumin seeds with ½ cup water, or enough to make a pestolike paste.
5. When the squash is cooked, add the ground coconut paste, the pinto beans, and the toasted coconut and cook for another 2 minutes; remove from the heat.

6. In a frying pan, heat the oil over medium-high heat. Add the mustard seeds and cover. When the seeds pop, toss in the dried red chilies and fry for a few seconds; then, if using, add the fresh curry leaves (watch for sputtering) and fry briefly until they finish crackling. Add the mixture to the squash and stir to combine.

SERVES 4 TO 6

THREE SOUTHERN SIDES

from Tamar Adler, chef of Farm255 in Athens, Georgia

"Our 'three sides' has been among our most popular dishes ever since it appeared on the menu and is in particular a favorite of a second-trimester mother-to-be," explains Adler. "The black-eyed peas, simply flavored with coconut milk, are the biggest hit. Incidentally, kids seem to love the dish, and even clear their plates of the greens, redolent of garlic as they are, and nestled up against the buttery mash."

TURNIP-POTATO MASH

3 pounds organic Yukon Gold or Cranberry Red potatoes
1 pound Purple Top White Globe or large Scarlet Queen turnips (or whichever
    variety is available)
Salt
4 tablespoons (½ stick) butter (organic/hormone-free/local)
2 cups half-and-half (organic/hormone-free/local)
Pepper

Scrub the potatoes, but do not peel. Cut the potatoes into sixths and the turnips into ½-inch pieces, as they are slightly harder than the potatoes but will cook at the same pace if cut into smaller pieces. Place the vegetables in a pot that accommodates them and leaves another good third of headspace, and cover with cold water by several inches. Salt the water liberally, cover, bring to a boil. Lower to a simmer once the pot is frothy, and simmer until the potatoes and turnips are easily pierced by a fork or become chalky when pinched with tongs. Just before the potatoes and turnips are ready, melt the butter in a small pan. Drain the vegetables in a large colander; tip the potatoes and turnips back into the cooking pot and add the melted butter and half-and-half and mash with a masher until well mixed but still exhibiting a little texture. Season with salt and pepper as desired.

SERVES 6 TO 8

BLACK-EYED PEAS

> 3 cups dried or canned organic black-eyed peas
> 1 to 2 tablespoons organic canola oil
> 3 cups diced yellow onions (Vidalia or other sweet variety, if available)
> 3 local tomatoes, blanched and peeled, or 3 to 4 canned whole peeled organic tomatoes, crushed against the sides of the can.
> Salt
> ½ can coconut milk
> ¼ cup finely chopped fresh cilantro

1. Soak the dried black-eyed peas at room temperature overnight in water to cover by 4 inches. The following day drain, and cook in cold water at a low simmer with no salt until cooked through and tender to the bite. Drain in a colander. If using canned, drain in a colander and rinse under cold running water.

2. In a pot, sauté the onions over low heat in the canola oil until they are releasing liquid; add the tomatoes and cook over low heat until integrated, 5 to 10 minutes. Add the peas and ½ can of the coconut milk and salt to taste; add more coconut milk if desired. When fully integrated, turn off the heat and mix the cilantro through the peas.

SERVES 6 TO 8

QUICK SAUTÉED GREENS

Any hearty greens (kale, chard, mustard, or turnip) will do, but we feel pretty strongly about the superiority of collards.

    2 pounds hearty greens, roughly cut into 2-inch-wide slices
    2 tablespoons olive oil
    Salt
    6 to 7 cloves garlic, sliced
    1 tablespoon to ¼ cup water
    Freshly squeezed lemon juice

Stem any greens with woody, fibrous stems except for chard (chard stems are often sweet). Heat the olive oil over medium heat. Add the hearty greens, a good couple of pinches of salt, and the garlic and toss until starting to wilt; add the water starting with 1 tablespoon, then adding more if your greens are dry, to finish cooking. Finish with a squeeze of fresh lemon.

SERVES 6 TO 8

FARM 255'S VERSION OF FANNIE FARMER'S RICH CORN CAKE

    1 cup organic Red Mule cornmeal (or other organic cornmeal)
    1 cup organic all-purpose flour
    3½ tablespoons sugar
    1 teaspoon baking soda
    2 teaspoons cream of tartar
    ¾ to 1 teaspoon salt (depending on your taste; we do a heavy ¾ teaspoon)
    1 cup full-fat organic sour cream
    ¼ cup full-fat organic milk
    2 organic eggs, well beaten
    4 tablespoons organic butter, melted
    1 tablespoon minced rosemary or sage (optional)

Preheat oven to 425 degrees F. Butter and flour (or spray with non-GMO, non-hydrogenated canola cooking spray) a 9-inch round baking tin. Combine cornmeal, flour, sugar, baking soda, cream of tartar, and salt and whisk together. Add all wet ingredients to cornmeal-flour mixture (sour cream, milk, beaten eggs, butter). Stir just until well combined, adding optional herbs along with wet ingredients if using. Tip into baking pan, using a spatula to spoon out all batter. Bake about 20 minutes. Cool and cut into slices to serve.

SERVE 6 TO 8

ALLEN FARM* CHICKEN WITH SPRING VEGETABLE RISOTTO

from Daniel Sauer, chef of the Outermost Inn on Martha's Vineyard, Massachusetts

"My wife Nonie became a very picky eater when she was pregnant with our first child. Before pregnancy, she had always been up for eating anything. But during her first trimester, she could stomach only chicken, bland vegetables, and starches. Pretty boring stuff for a chef to cook. We found going back to basics to be a simple solution for both of us. She could keep them down and I found real pleasure in cooking nutritious meals for my unborn child. This chicken recipe using local, organic produce became one of her absolute favorites."

1 large chicken, about 4 pounds (trussed for roasting)
8 cups chicken stock
3 tablespoons extra-virgin olive oil

Clarissa Allen and Mitchell Posen are seasoned island farmers with a passion for sustainable, organic agriculture and livestock. We use their chicken for this recipe.

2 tablespoons butter

2 cups carnaroli or arborio rice

1 cup dry white wine

1 cup minced spring onions

½ cup shelled peas

½ cup shelled fava beans

½ cup thin asparagus (cut into ¼-inch pieces)

1 tablespoon fresh flat parley (chopped)

1 tablespoon mint (chopped)

½ cup grated pasteurized parmesan cheese

Salt and pepper to taste

1. Place large stock pot of water on stove and bring to a boil. Season water with salt.
2. Preheat oven to 375 degrees F. Season chicken with salt and pepper and place it in a roasting pan. Roast chicken uncovered, basting every 15 minutes until internal temperature reaches 165 degrees F for approximately 15 to 18 minutes per pound. Allow bird to rest (for redistribution of juices). Once cool, remove legs and thighs. Pull meat from legs and thighs and discard bones and skin. Set meat aside for use in risotto.
3. While bird is roasting or resting, set up a bowl of ice water next to your pot of boiling water. Place the shelled peas in the boiling water until tender (the best way to check if a vegetable is tender is to taste it). Remove quickly and blanch (place in ice bath to stop the cooking process). Repeat with the fava beans and the asparagus separately. This is an important step that will keep the vegetables bright and retain their flavor. Also please note that favas will have to peeled again after being blanched.
4. Bring stock to a simmer. Heat 1 tablespoon of olive oil and 1 tablespoon of butter in deep heavy sauté pan. Stir in onions and cook over medium heat until translucent but not browned. Add rice and stir continuously for 4 minutes. Do not allow rice to brown. Add wine and cook over medium heat until rice has absorbed all of the liquid. Add 2 cups of hot stock and again stir until absorbed. Add another 2 cups of stock and stir until absorbed. Repeat step until rice is cooked but still al dente, about 18 to 20 minutes. Stir in thigh meat

and vegetables. Remove from heat and stir in cheese, remaining tablespoon of butter, parsley and mint. Add salt and pepper to taste. Serve with the remaining chicken.

SERVES 4

CORN SOUP WITH GRILLED FLORIDA PRAWNS AND YELLOW GRIT TIMBALE

from Bradley Ogden, chef/partner of Bradley Ogden, Caesars Palace, Las Vegas, Nevada, co-founder and co-proprietor of the nine-restaurant Lark Creek Restaurant Group, and long-time organic devotee

This was the "last supper" for some regular guests of Chef Bradley Ogden. "They were sitting on the patio at Lark Creek underneath the redwoods, she ate this, and she went into labor the next morning," he says. Ogden is unaware if it has had similar effect for other women but thinks it probably has. "Maybe over the thousands of people I have cooked for." To keep this dish as organic as possible, try to get fresh prawns in season from someone you trust.

SOUP

2 tablespoons unsalted butter

2 tablespoons seeded and minced poblano pepper

1 cup yellow Spanish onion, peeled and cut into ½-inch dice

4 ounces Yukon Gold or white creamer potatoes, washed and scrubbed, skin left on, cut into ½-inch dice and rinsed in cold water

5 cups fresh corn kernels

4 cups corn stock (see below)

2 teaspoons fresh ground black pepper

1 tablespoon olive oil

12 fresh Florida prawns, peeled and deveined, or other fresh prawns

Add the butter to a wide, 8-quart, heavy-bottomed saucepan and place over medium heat. Add the chile, onion, and potatoes. Season lightly with salt and pepper. Cover and sweat for 8 minutes, stirring occasionally. Add the corn, cover again, and cook for another 10 minutes, stirring often. Add the stock, cover, and gently simmer for 15 minutes. Adjust seasoning with salt and pepper. Remove from the heat and lightly cool. Puree in a food processor or blender and strain. If too thick, adjust consistency with a little more corn stock. If not using immediately, cool soup over an ice bath.

SERVES 4 TO 6

CORN STOCK

10 yellow or white corncobs, chopped into 2-inch pieces

3 cups corn kernels

3 medium carrots, peeled and chopped

1 white onion, peeled and chopped

2 celery stalks, chopped

6 cloves garlic, peeled

¼ cup finely sliced lemongrass

½ bay leaf

12 parsley stems

1 tablespoon peppercorns

Combine all the ingredients in a large stainless steel stockpot. Cover ingredients with water over high heat, and bring to a boil. Reduce heat and simmer slowly for 45 minutes. Remove from the heat. Strain through a fine mesh strainer and cool in an ice bath. When the stock is cool, transfer it to a storage container and refrigerate until needed. If freezing, store in 1-cup containers.

MAKES 5 CUPS

Grilled Florida Prawns and Yellow Grit Timbale

12 fresh Florida prawns, or other fresh prawns
1/2 cup uncooked yellow corn grits
3/4 cup milk
1 cup heavy cream
1/2 teaspoon minced garlic
3/4 teaspoon kosher salt
1/4 teaspoon fresh cracked black pepper
2 eggs
1 pinch nutmeg
1 tablespoon unsalted butter

1. Grill the prawns, shells on, over hot coals for 2 minutes. The prawns should be slightly undercooked. Let cool. Peel, devein, and chop into 1/2-inch pieces.
2. Preheat oven to 300 degrees F. Butter six 3-ounce timbale molds.
3. In a small saucepan, combine the grits, milk, 1/4 cup of the cream, garlic, and 1/4 teaspoon of the salt and pepper. Simmer slowly, covered, over low heat, for 15 minutes. Remove from the heat, uncover, and cool.
4. In a small bowl, mix together the remaining cream and 1/2 teaspoon of salt, eggs, and nutmeg. Place 2 tablespoons of cooked grits in each mold. Divide the chopped prawns evenly between the molds. Fill to the top with the custard mixture. Place in a water bath and bake in the oven for 20 minutes or until set. Let cool slightly before removing from timbale molds.

To serve: Heat the soup. While the soup is reheating, grill the 12 prawns over hot coals. Unmold the grit timbale and place it, top side up, in the center of a large soup plate. Pour 6 ounces of soup around the timbale and arrange 3 grilled prawns per serving.

SERVES 4 TO 6

CLASSIC BEEF STEW

from Mark Bittman, New York Times *food columnist and best selling author of* How to Cook Everything

. . . .

Stew might be the most comforting of comfort foods. It's also brimming with things a pregnant woman needs—protein, iron, vegetables. But the best part—especially for parents who already have a young kid and one on the way—is that it lasts. Make one pot and eat it over the course of a week. The luxury of not cleaning or cooking for those few days could be as beneficial as the carrots.

Browning the beef before braising adds another dimension of flavor, but isn't absolutely necessary. Try it both ways; skipping the browning step saves time and mess.

> 2 tablespoons canola or other neutral oil, or olive oil
> 1 clove garlic, lightly crushed, plus 1 tablespoon minced garlic
> 2 to 2½ pounds beef chuck or round, trimmed of surface fat and cut into 1- to
>   1½-inch cubes
> Salt and freshly ground black pepper to taste
> 2 large or 3 medium onions, cut into eighths
> 3 tablespoons flour
> 3 cups chicken, beef, or vegetable stock, or water, or wine, or a combination
> 1 bay leaf
> 1 teaspoon fresh thyme leaves or ½ teaspoon dried thyme
> 4 medium-to-large potatoes, peeled and cut into 1-inch chunks
> 4 large carrots, peeled and cut into 1-inch chunks
> 1 cup fresh or frozen (thawed) peas
> Minced fresh parsley leaves for garnish

1. Heat a large casserole or deep skillet that can later be covered over medium-high heat for 2 to 3 minutes; add the oil and the crushed garlic clove; cook, stirring for 1 minute, then remove and discard the garlic. Add the meat chunks to the skillet a few at a time, turning to brown well on all sides. Do not crowd or they will not brown properly; cook them in batches if necessary.

(You may find it easier to do the initial browning in the oven: Preheat to 500 degrees F and roast the meat with 1 tablespoon of the oil and the garlic clove, shaking the pan to turn them once or twice, until brown all over. Remove the garlic clove before continuing.) Season the meat with salt and pepper as it cooks.

2. When the meat is brown, remove it with a slotted spoon. Pour or spoon off most of the fat and turn the heat to medium. Add the onions. Cook, stirring until they soften, about 10 minutes. Add the flour and cook, stirring for about 2 minutes. Add the stock or water or wine, bay leaf, thyme, and meat, and bring to a boil. Turn the heat to low and cover. Cook undisturbed for 30 minutes.

3. Uncover the pan; the mixture should be quite soupy (if it is not, add a little more liquid). Add the potatoes and carrots, turn the heat up for a minute or so to resume boiling, then lower the heat and cover again. Cook 30 to 60 minutes until the meat and vegetables are tender. Taste for seasoning and add more salt, pepper, and/or thyme if necessary. (If you are not planning to serve the stew immediately, remove the meat and vegetables with a slotted spoon and refrigerate them and the stock separately. Skim the fat from the stock before combining it with the meat and vegetables, reheating, and proceeding with the recipe from this point.)

4. Add the minced garlic and the peas; if you are pleased with the stew's consistency, continue to cook covered over low heat. If it is too soupy, remove the cover and raise the heat to high. In either case, cook an additional 5 minutes or so, until the peas have heated through and the garlic flavor has pervaded the stew. Garnish and serve.

SERVES 4 TO 6

TIME: 1½ TO 2 HOURS, LARGELY UNATTENDED

PICKLES

PICKLED OKRA

from Peter Hoffman, chef of Savoy Restaurant in New York City

. . . .

"Caribbean folklore is that okra helps the baby come on and starts labor. My wife decided that she had had enough of being pregnant the second time around, so she ate a big jar of pickled okra (she also took some castor oil, which certainly didn't hurt), and she started her labor fast and furious," recalls Hoffman. "One hour, to be exact. And I delivered the baby on the front steps of our apartment."

> 1 pound small okra pods (cut off any darkened stems but leave whole)
> 3 cloves garlic, halved
> 1 cup cider vinegar
> 1 cup rice wine vinegar
> 1 cup water
> 3 tablespoons kosher salt
> ½ teaspoon dried red pepper flakes
> 2 teaspoons mustard seeds
> 1 teaspoon dill seeds

Pack three 1-pint canning jars with the okra vertical and alternating stems and tips. Put a halved garlic clove in each jar as well. In a nonreactive metal pot, bring the liquids to a boil. Add the salt and spices. Allow to steep for 20 minutes. Fill the jars with the liquid to within 1 inch of the rims. Wipe the rims and put on the lids. Put the glass jars on a rack in a deep kettle and cover with hot water by 2 inches. Bring to a boil, cover, and boil for 10 minutes. Remove the jars from the bath and leave to cool. Let the pickles mellow for 2 weeks minimum before tasting. Best at 1 month.

MAKES 3 PINTS

ICE CREAM

MULBERRY ICE CREAM

from Alice Waters, author, food activist, and chef/founder of Chez Panisse in Berkeley, California

. . . .

"There is no question I just wanted ice cream," Waters recalls of being pregnant with her daughter, Fanny. "I ate it at the restaurant. I couldn't pass an ice cream place without wanting to stop. I just had a terrible craving."

9 egg yolks
1½ cups half-and-half
1¾ cups sugar
3 cups heavy cream
3 cups mulberries
2 tablespoons lemon juice
1 tablespoon kirsch

1. Whisk the egg yolks in a mixing bowl just enough to break them up. Gently heat the half-and-half and 1 cup of the sugar in a nonreactive saucepan, stirring slowly over low heat until the half-and-half is steaming and the sugar is dissolved. Drizzle the warm sweetened half-and-half into the egg yolks, whisking constantly as you pour.
2. Return the mixture to the saucepan. Cook over low heat, stirring and scraping the bottom of the pan with a wooden spoon or a heat-resistant rubber spatula, until the mixture is thick enough to coat the spoon. Immediately remove from the heat and strain through a fine-mesh sieve into a bowl with the heavy cream. Chill thoroughly.
3. Stir together the berries and the remaining ¾ cup sugar in a nonreactive saucepan over medium heat until the sugar dissolves and the berries begin to release their juice. Puree the berries in a food processor and pass through the sieve. Stir the berry mixture into the chilled ice cream base. Stir in the lemon

juice and kirsch. Freeze according to the instructions for your ice cream maker.

MAKES 3 PINTS

BABY FOOD

HOMEMADE ORGANIC BABY FOOD

from Moon Unit Zappa, writer, comic, and filmmaker

. . . .

What you'll need:

1. A list of approved foods from your pediatrician, which will tell you all the foods babies can eat and in what order and at what ages. The list should also include what reactions to watch for.
2. Once you have that list, first try some of the organic jarred stuff to figure out what your baby likes. My kick-ass friend Michelle said to check with your market or health food store to see if you can get discounts for buying your organic baby food in bulk. Do! You will want to have some of the jarred stuff in your pantry in case of emergency, exhaustion, or spontaneous outings with friends. I always keep a few jars on hand in my diaper bag in case I decide to have a sudden adventure with my sweet baby.
3. Invest in some kind of device that grinds food up, like a potato ricer or a hand grinder and/or something else that can puree stuff. I use my Cuisinart for the pureeing, and my $8 food mill for everything else. You can always use your blender or food processor for the pureeing, but a portable hand grinder or baby-food mill comes in extra handy when you want to go to lunch and you don't want to bring any jarred stuff along.
4. Food cube trays (preferably not plastic).
5. Lots of shatterproof glass containers for storage.

6. Lastly, invest in *Super Baby Food* by Ruth Yaron. She has written the quintessential book on what babies eat, and although it's three knuckles' worth of more information than you might need, her epic tome on the subject is a lifesaver!

How to make organic baby food:

1. Buy the organic, pesticide-free version of the approved food on your doc's list from your local health food store or farmers' market.
2. Cook it to your baby's preferred consistency in your preferred cooking style (steam, bake, boil, microwave), and reserve some of the cooking water if applicable. Chop veggies into miniature cubes and place in a frying pan with a little bit of water, then cover and combo steam/boil/stir-fry it before mashing it in the food mill or pureeing it with a little of the reserved cooking water.
3. Stick the puree in food cube trays and pop it in the freezer. The next day, transfer the cubes to individual glass containers with one or two or three cubes in each, date the containers, and pop them back in the freezer.
4. Come mealtime, heat the individual portion, and, voilà! Watch your baby smile, and enjoy knowing that you are making a huge difference in your baby's health, life, and future!

ACKNOWLEDGMENTS

Tamar Adler
Susan Allport
Dan Barber
Gregor Barnum
Kirstin Binder
Mark Bittman
Kimberly Brown
Edward Burlingame
Perdita Burlingame
Roger Burlingame
Susan Burton
Leah Carlson-Stanisic
Olli Chanoff
Tara Cibelli
Theo Colborn
Consumer Reports
Annette Corkey
Corrina
Debra Lynn Dadd
Brendan Dolan
Siobhan Dolan
Michelle Dominguez
Susan Eng

Tim Fitzgerald
Ben Ford
Holly Givens
Myra Goodman
Google
Hallie Greider
Joan Dye Gussow
Irene Hamburger
Lisa Hamilton
Harriet
Amanda Hesser
Jack Hitt
Peter Hoffman
Kathryn Huck-Seymour
Alexandra Jacobs
Laura Just
Maya Kaimal
Deb Kavakos
Barbara Kingsolver
Julie Klam
Pamela Koch
Stacey Koff
Terri Kurtzberg

Susan West Kurz
Angie Lee
George Leonard
Jo Lipstadt
Deborah Madison
Danielle Mattoon
David McCormick
Bill Meaders
Marcella Melandri
Christie Mellor
Victoria Misrock
Julie Torres Moskovitz
Marion Nestle
Catherine Newman
Mara Lopez Nishita
Bradley Ogden
Mary Ellen O'Neill
Mindy Pennybacker
Michael Pollan
Kate Porterfield
Nora Poullion
Jessica Prentice
Miranda Purves

Amy Redfern
Andrea Rosen
Lisa Sanders
Daniel Sauer
Wenonah Madison Sauer
Erika Schreder
Sally Schultheiss
Ruth Shalit
Kate Sharp
Anne Singer
Ryu Spaeth
Joe Tessitore
Amy Vreeland
Janette Wallis
Alice Waters
Amanda White
Florence Williams
Ali Wing
Beth Wishnie
Moon Unit Zappa
Aili Chanoff Zissu
Roger Zissu
Suzanne Zissu

INDEX